Health Facility
Commissioning
GUIDELINES

Health Facility
Commissioning
GUIDELINES

Quality through Collaboration

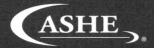

THE AMERICAN SOCIETY FOR HEALTHCARE ENGINEERING
OF THE AMERICAN HOSPITAL ASSOCIATION

CHICAGO

The American Society for Healthcare Engineering
of the American Hospital Association
155 North Wacker Drive, Suite 400
Chicago, IL 60606
312-422-3800
ashe@aha.org
www.ashe.org

Dale Woodin, CHFM, FASHE, Executive Director
Douglas S. Erickson, FASHE, CHFM, HFDP, CHC, Deputy Executive Director
Patrick J. Andrus, Director, Business Development
Pamela James Blumgart, Senior Editor
Susan G. Rubin, MPH, Senior Specialist, Marketing & Communications

Cover photographs: Vista Award winners from 2006 and 2009 (an awards program sponsored by
ASHE and the AIA Academy of Architecture for Health)
  ◆ Exterior and drawing elevation, Integrated Research Center, St. Jude's Children's Research
    Hospital, Memphis, Tennessee
  ◆ Boiler and generator, Fairbanks Memorial Hospital/Denali Center, Fairbanks, Alaska
  ◆ Operating room, SSM Cardinal Glennon Children's Medical Center, St. Louis, Missouri
Additional photo credits: Two businessmen shaking hands: Cimmerian © iStock, Teamwork:
LajosRepasi © iStock.

ISBN: 978-0-87258-873-8
ASHE catalog #: 055380

Printed in the United States of America on archival quality paper
Design by www.DesignForBooks.com

First printing: June 2010
Second printing: November 2010

Contents

CHAPTER 4: TRANSITION TO OPERATIONAL SUSTAINABILITY 53

CHAPTER 5: POSTOCCUPANCY AND WARRANTY PHASE 65

CHAPTER 6: RETROCOMMISSIONING 71

APPENDICES 77

Preface

Throughout its life cycle, a modern health care facility will be met with changing occupancies, additional regulatory requirements, opportunities to upgrade technologies and efficiencies, and constantly evolving patient care, education, and research missions. To stay abreast of developments in the industry, health care organizations must carefully maintain and constantly refresh their facilities. When owners identify the need for a change, they engage professional designers and contractors to develop their concepts into structures, which the health care organization then owns and operates to meet the needs of its business.

Despite many changes in the approach to health care design and construction, health care organizations' desire to achieve a suitable return on investment (ROI) from their facility projects has remained a relatively low priority for most project teams. A major obstacle to turning this situation around has been continuation of the interdisciplinary silos that have long existed throughout the facility life cycle continuum, from project inception through operation and maintenance of a completed facility. These silos interfere with collaboration among project participants that could improve the project team's ability to optimize the health care physical environment.

The ASHE health facility commissioning (HFCx) process introduced in these guidelines is designed to provide the project delivery team with a robust set of tools to help improve initial project commissioning collaboration, continuing commissioning behaviors, and retrocommissioning tactics. The guidelines will assist facility professionals in their efforts to optimize the health care physical environment while achieving the ROI their organizations desire from their projects.

The introduction of this broader, more collaborative commissioning process may be met with some resistance, but change must happen to ensure a health care organization's best interests are met in all phases of the facility life cycle. When told their buildings require extra air exchanges, stringently controlled temperature and humidity, high color-rendering lighting, and sophisticated electrical distribution and backup systems, owners fund the work in the belief that the professionals they have engaged will optimize their investments. However, without project commissioning and a team focus on the full life cycle cost, the desired ROI is not guaranteed and generally not obtained. Protecting the owner's ROI should be one of the primary purposes of health care facility professionals as they deliver a project that meets the owner's project requirements.

Proper commissioning is only one factor in reaching the owner's desired ROI from a project. First cost is also important, and commissioning will ensure a facility design does not create unnecessary first cost or value reduction from value engineering (VE) exercises. (Many refer to the VE process as "value eradication" because it can, if not used properly, reduce rather than increase project value.) Additional factors contributing to the ROI goal are owning and operating costs. These expenses and savings begin when the owner takes productive use of a facility, and they can have a profound impact on project performance. Because the O&M team is often given only a cursory role in the project delivery process, team members only get involved when a new or renovated project is completed and they take over its operation and maintenance. Without early involvement in a project, extensive training in efficient equipment and systems operation, and a clear understanding of the purposes of the health facility commissioning process, it is very difficult for the O&M team to balance the competing agendas of maintaining high customer service levels and focusing on the commissioning authority's effort to obtain the ROI. These competing agendas have strong messages and the owner will not waver on either, which is what makes commissioning so important to health care projects.

It is time to broaden the scope of standard operating procedures in health care facility project management to make commissioning a normal part of every health facility project, regardless of project size or cost. ASHE is convinced that health facility commissioning is critical to the success of every project, and we anticipate these guidelines will bridge the gaps between the efforts of various stakeholders throughout a facility's life cycle. This belief and our commitment to "optimizing the health care physical environment" were the genesis for the development of the ASHE *Health Facility Commissioning Guidelines*.

There are many excellent commissioning processes and guidelines in the marketplace already, but none of them specifically addresses the complexities of commissioning health care facilities. It was with this knowledge and after due diligence and research into existing products that the ASHE Research and Development Committee prioritized the goal of developing the HFCx guidelines to complement the ASHE construction product portfolio. These guidelines are the first part of an ASHE HFCx lineup that will include a handbook, training for health care executives and facility professionals, and a health facility commissioning certification to be developed over the next few years. It is with this commitment that ASHE has developed these guidelines to support its members in their quest to bring home the ROI from their commissioning activities.

Development of these guidelines required much effort over many months. The draft was written by the following ASHE members:

Mark Kenneday, MBA, CHFM, SASHE
    Vice Chancellor, Campus Operations, University of Arkansas
    for Medical Sciences

Steven R. "Rusty" Ross, PE, LEED AP BD+C, CxA
    Vice President, Director of Commissioning Services,
    Smith Seckman Reid, Inc.

R. Clay Seckman, PE
    Executive Vice President, Smith Seckman Reid, Inc.

Ed Tinsley, PE, CEM, LEED AP, HFDP
    Managing Principal/Chairman of the Board, TME, Inc.

We would like to thank the following individuals for taking the time to review and comment on the draft document: Mike Locke; Damian Skelton, MBA, PE, CHFM; Kenneth A. Monroe, PE; Yeqiao Zhu, PhD, PE, CEM, LEED AP; Tyson K. Glimme, QCxP; Timothy M. Peglow, PE, MBA, MSE; Capt. Keith Shortall, PE; and Tim Staley, PE, CEM, LEED AP, HFDP, GBE.

Finally, we would like to thank the ASHE staff for their support of our effort.

Mark Kenneday
Rusty Ross
Clay Seckman
Ed Tinsley
May 2010

PART I

An Introduction
to Health Facility
Commissioning

These ASHE health facility commissioning guidelines were created to provide a commissioning process structured to meet the specific needs of the health care industry. The guidelines provide a standard set of terms, definitions, and processes. The consistency these standards can bring to the process of commissioning health care facilities will facilitate a project team's ability to deliver projects with an optimal return on investment (ROI).

While other commissioning guidelines exist, none is written specifically for the health care environment. It is critical that the process used for commissioning health care facilities accommodate the unique challenges of their specialized systems and function. The ASHE commissioning process, hereinafter referred to as health facility commissioning (HFCx), is also unique in that the entire project team, along with the commissioning authority, is accountable for actual building performance.

These guidelines are intended to establish a standard language and process for commissioning health care facilities that are cost-effective and efficient and that deliver the desired ROI. The guidelines can be adopted into construction and maintenance bid documents to ensure respondents have clear and concise definitions and instructions for formulating their estimates. The guidelines will remove ambiguity and inconsistencies in commissioning language and process, optimizing the ability of health care organizations to obtain accurate and effective pricing for their health care projects.

WHAT IS HEALTH FACILITY COMMISSIONING?

As is true for many terms used to define improved construction-related activities, the word "commissioning" often means something different to different people depending on their education, background, and training. For the purpose of these guidelines, the word "commissioning" means a process intended to ensure that building systems are installed and perform in accordance with the design intent, that the design intent is consistent with the owner's project requirements, and that operations and maintenance staff are adequately prepared to operate and maintain the completed facility. Additional language in the guidelines properly defines related activities that support the HFCx process.

Achieving desired outcomes from the HFCx process requires a clear definition of individual roles and responsibilities.

Achieving desired outcomes from the HFCx process requires a clear definition of individual roles and responsibilities. The owner should designate a health facility commissioning authority (HFCxA) who will manage the commissioning process. The HFCxA should be a qualified representative of the owner or an independent third party. The commissioning activities are allocated between the owner, the contractor, the design team, and the HFCxA. Once the commissioning team has been created, it should be empowered with the authority to work with the project team to meet the commissioning goals and the owner's project requirements.

For optimal outcomes, the HFCx team should be established and engaged at the outset of a project and remain fully involved throughout the planning, design, and construction process. This early involvement will optimize the effectiveness of the commissioning process and result in the greatest ROI.

By contrast, value engineering exercises are usually a knee-jerk reaction to a problem with project cost or schedule. Seldom do these activities result in true value-added solutions, and they generally save only a fraction of the actual cost. By contrast, a fully empowered HFCx team can develop value-added solutions that will reduce initial cost by providing effective alternatives early in the design process that do not compromise the owner's project requirements.

WHAT COMMISSIONING MEANS TO THE C-LEVEL

"C-level" is a term that describes the leadership team of a health care facility—generally a chief executive officer, chief operating officer, chief financial officer, chief nursing officer, and others with similar titles. Due to differences in education, training, and perspective, the C-level frequently speaks a vastly different language than the health care facility management professional. Frequently, this language barrier prevents effective communication of the value of commissioning, which may result in an uninformed decision by the C-level to remove the funds needed to support effective commissioning from a project budget.

To successfully campaign for scarce capital to properly fund sustained commissioning, health care facility management professionals must develop their business acumen to better fit the value expectations and financial models used by the C-level. The facility management culture must align with the mission and vision of the health care organization and support quality patient care, education, research, and community outreach. Properly commissioning projects is not sufficient to accomplish this. After taking over a new or renovated facility, the operations team must support behaviors that will ensure optimal outcomes over time. Selling the C-level on how commissioning can facilitate both satisfactory design and installation of new equipment and optimal operations over time is vital to acquiring proper funding.

One of the greatest challenges for any project is cost management. Planning, design, and construction (PDC) project costs are generally not well understood by the executive team, and they usually do not have a great deal of experiential data on which to base comparisons. Health care facility management professionals must do a better job of developing the business case and value equation to support commissioning activities. To reduce anxiety and ensure the process is not driven solely on cost, the benefits of commissioning must be properly identified and marketed to the C-level.

The value derived from commissioning activities can be shown as a simple relationship in which the benefit obtained from commissioning is divided by the cost to deliver it. The relationship at the core of this discussion is this:

$$Value = Benefits/Cost$$

The greater the benefit derived from a specific cost, the greater the value to leadership. Therefore, a primary objective is to document and communicate the value the C-level derives from properly commissioning a project: Commissioning lowers the cost of constructing and operating a health care facility, delivering exceptional value. For a project to deliver the highest value, it is essential for it to be fully commissioned.

The contract administration services provided by the design team should not be mistaken for commissioning. Contract administration requires only a general familiarity with the work and provides for documentation only of deficiencies that are obvious or discovered through random sampling or contractor testing. Although these services complement the commissioning process, they are distinctly different from commissioning activities. Contract administration notes deficiencies, but does not document items that were installed or operating correctly at the time of occupancy. The commissioning process documents system performance and functionality in accordance with the owner's project requirements while noting all deficiencies from the contract documents.

Benchmarking documentation of equipment installation and performance is the fundamental element of commissioning that separates this process from contract administration services and the construction process. Commissioning provides a comprehensive record of what systems were reviewed over

The greater the benefit derived from a specific cost, the greater the value to leadership.

the course of the project. Contract administration, on the other hand, only assumes that all systems have been reviewed. In fact, standard AIA documents only require the design team to be "generally familiar" with the work installed.

In addition to its other services, commissioning optimizes costs in all phases of a project. It is proactive and identifies potential problems and conflicts from the design phase through the occupancy phase, including before the design is finalized and before construction phase issues affect the construction schedule or become operational issues. Commissioning reduces change orders, requests for information (RFIs), schedule delays, deficiencies at substantial completion, and postoccupancy O&M man-hours after the facility has been occupied. The impact of not engaging in commissioning is the cost associated with problems not discovered, design issues revealed after the bid process, system operational issues that occur postoccupancy, building pressurization issues that create infiltration problems that can lead to mold, and so on.

Proper commissioning operations can provide additional value over time. ROI in a health care project depends on the successful execution of two strategies: The first is optimizing space utility and project cost and achieving installed systems that perform as intended from a construction or renovation project. The second is safe, efficient, cost-effective operation of the completed project or facility for its intended purpose. Making ongoing commissioning and support of commissioning behaviors an integral component of the health care facility management culture will help ensure these strategies are successful and sustainable.

The value obtained from a properly commissioned project can quickly evaporate as a result of incompatible maintenance practices. Consequently, the C-level marketing plan should include change initiatives that support ongoing activities related to the commissioning directive as well as the initial cost of the commissioning effort. The full value of commissioning cannot be realized unless operations and maintenance activities have been structured to maintain system performance at optimum levels. Absent this emphasis, the performance of the commissioned systems will erode over time.

THE COMMISSIONING BUSINESS PLAN

It is important to recognize that the audience of a request to fund a health care commissioning project is generally not a group of engineers, architects, contractors, or facility personnel. In most cases, the audience is business professionals trained to make sound business decisions based on health-related information, scientific research, heath education-based arguments, and administrative requirements presented by the medical staff, clinicians, researchers, and academicians who constitute the core mission and support staff of the institution. Their experience, education, and business training prepare these business pro-

It is important to recognize that the audience of a request to fund a health care commissioning project is generally not a group of engineers, architects, contractors, or facility personnel.

fessionals to evaluate the HFCx proposal on its mission-specific and financial merits. Like most industries, the health care industry has many standard protocols that must be included in a successful project proposal. The most important of these is the development and presentation of a business plan.

The first thing to remember when developing a business plan for commissioning is that every initiative and project proposal is in competition for scarce resources. These resources can be reduced to three primary concerns—people, materials, and cash. There is also the issue of time, which is not a concrete resource, but must be managed in conjunction with the resource groups. The fact that these resources are scarce should not be forgotten, and a successful business plan will always treat them as rare and hard to come by.

Once capital resources have been allocated to a project, the focus should shift from competition for capital to optimizing project performance as C-level expectations are now at peak levels. Keeping the scarcity of resources in focus is the responsibility of the project executive sponsor, who should serve as the champion for resource management and prudence. For a health facility commissioning project, this responsibility generally falls to the executive who is over the facilities department. Depending on the business model and size of the institution, facilities may be a single department that represents design, construction, and O&M or separate, more process-specific departments. Whatever the model or size of the institution, it is imperative that the executive consider all these resources along with the material and financial requirements for a successful commissioning outcome.

Using an accepted convention to develop a business plan will result in a standard product that is familiar to its readers. As with most standards, deviation creates confusion and may not garner the acceptance desired. Accountants use generally accepted principles (GAP) that dictate a format and process for assuring uniformity of financial reporting. In construction project delivery, Construction Specifications Institute (CSI) divisions are used to document the scope. In financial markets, investment vehicles are used to reduce risk while growing wealth. In the business community, a business plan is used to develop a proposal, grow support, obtain approval, and implement the plan. Business plans that follow this protocol are much more likely to meet with success, although the quality and content of the argument is still the primary motivator for funding.

A great business plan cannot significantly improve a poorly positioned campaign, but health facility commissioning is almost always an easy campaign to wage on its virtue and it is generally easy to document a significant ROI. A great business plan makes the argument that much better, improving the odds that HFCx projects will be funded and successful. The challenge is to present the argument in a manner that is concise and clear to business decision-makers.

Using an accepted convention to develop a business plan will result in a standard product that is familiar to its readers.

A business plan has eight parts that are routinely presented in this order:

1. Executive summary and table of contents
2. Current plan
3. SWOT analysis
4. Goals
5. Business strategies
6. New service programs
7. Financial projections
8. Quality controls

Each section describes an important aspect of the plan and should be developed in the order shown to ensure continuity of thought and recognition of the circumstances surrounding the proposal. A great commissioning project should be supported by a business plan that fully develops the opportunity it offers and the likelihood of its success.

Executive Summary

The executive summary should summarize the project and present the HFCx opportunity in simple business terms. Consideration should be given to the executive's schedule and volume of reading when developing the summary. A good executive summary is never more than a page, and a great summary is generally a half page in length. Assume the attention span of the average health care executive does not exceed 15 to 20 seconds. If material does not grab his or her attention or speak to a specific need the organization has been trying to fill, the executive will not read it through.

Because most executives are acutely aware of the utility cost to operate their facility and the cost of construction-related activities, the summary in a commissioning business plan should focus on the opportunity to reduce the first cost of the project and to support operational sustainability that will ensure long-term ROI is derived once the project is in service. The summary should also make clear the improved reliability of systems that have been commissioned. As well, the executive summary is an excellent place to explain how a fully commissioned project and the health facility commissioning team contribute not only to safe and effective delivery of the project but to improving the daily operations of the health care facility. All of these arguments should be made in the context of how they will improve patient care, education, and research and support the core mission of the institution.

The table of contents should include the standard eight sections of the business plan, with only minor changes from project to project. This approach

The executive summary should summarize the project and present the HFCx opportunity in simple business terms.

will create consistency in the team's efforts, aiding future business plan development and standardizing the team's presentations. Over time, the priorities of the executive team will become clear and the table of contents can be targeted to better meet their expectations.

Current Plan

The section on the current plan is the place to provide the executive team or C-suite with an accurate picture of the present situation. The best approach is to give them a snapshot of what currently happens when you facilitate a project. For new construction, a description of how the project would be delivered without the HFCx process is a good approach. Outcomes should be included that enumerate the financial and operating parameters sought and obtained using current strategies and objectives. If there is a clear objective such as achieving an Energy Star rating, be sure to mention it and show the metrics used to assess whether the objective has been achieved.

This is not the time to embellish problems associated with the current plan, but rather to identify what is normally done. It is appropriate to note what works well and what the limitations of the current process are. Be careful not to disparage the current plan as it has served the institution well and may be the legacy of a member of the C-suite.

SWOT Analysis

An effective business plan always includes a SWOT (strengths, weaknesses, opportunities, and threats) analysis. This covers both macro- and microeconomic business factors that have been analyzed to better understand their effect on the outcome of the proposed business plan. The best SWOT analysis for a HFCx project will include factors both internal and external to the institution. The strengths and weaknesses of the plan and business unit should reflect the risks associated with specific opportunities and threats in the community, such as volatile utility rates and adverse changes in utility reliability. The C-suite should be assured that all factors were evaluated and the project team understands and considered their impact on the success of the initiative. When resources are very tight, this reassurance can be the difference between a funded HFCx project and one that is placed on hold for a more opportune time. During the presentation, the C-level executives usually ask questions about the factors considered that will affect the success of the project. A quick answer and reference to the SWOT analysis will ensure proper navigation of this hurdle.

Goals

In this section, the goals of the plan are outlined. This is where the overarching outcomes sought from the initiative are identified. It is imperative to clearly spell out what costs and benefits can be derived from a HFCx project so the C-suite can begin to frame their value equation.

In developing commissioning goals, it is sometimes helpful to consider goals the C-suite would want to address, such as patient safety, increased market share, space utilization, ROI, safe staffing levels, reduced infection rates, and patient and visitor satisfaction. Business goals should always be expressed in terms of customer-defined value. In the case of commissioning, this is the value the customer—both internal and external—will derive from the commissioning project.

The health care executive reading the business plan is primarily motivated by projects that will enhance and grow the core competencies of the institution, especially patient care, education, and research. Be sure to define how the HFCx project will directly support the growth of these business imperatives. For example:

> A properly commissioned HVAC system in surgery will ensure better defined levels of temperature and humidity, which will translate into lower surgical site and other nosocomial infections. The lower rate of infection will decrease the number of return cases and improve surgery throughput as well as support marketing of high-quality, low-"incidence of occurrence" invasive procedures. An additional incentive is the reduced kWh consumption rate achieved when properly commissioned equipment operates at peak efficiency levels and provides the responsiveness needed to maintain finite temperature variations critical to cardiovascular procedures that require use of a heart/lung bypass machine.

Once goals have been defined, the next step is to reverse-engineer the strategies and objectives required to achieve those goals. Using this method, the strategies developed are what need to be done to achieve the desired goals, and the objectives provide indicators for measuring the success of the project.

Business Strategies

The next section outlines business strategies for achieving the goals of the HFCx project. Include a brief explanation of the strategies that will be employed to achieve each HFCx goal. These strategies will be better defined in the next section, but because it is important for the executive to see that the goals are supported by responsible strategies and objectives, it is a good idea to introduce them here.

Be sure to include a description of the support that will be needed from various departments in the health care organization (e.g., accounting, facilities, design and construction, administration) as well as from supporting consultants.

To ensure a HFCx project campaign is properly prioritized and has the best chance of receiving funding, its goals and strategies must be clearly stated in terms that business professionals understand and supported by responsible measures of success. Each objective must be measurable and important enough to count.

HFCx project goals are well-suited to the use of management-by-objectives (MBO) strategies. For example, a typical MBO strategy for the goal of achieving continuous commissioning might look like that shown in Figure 1.

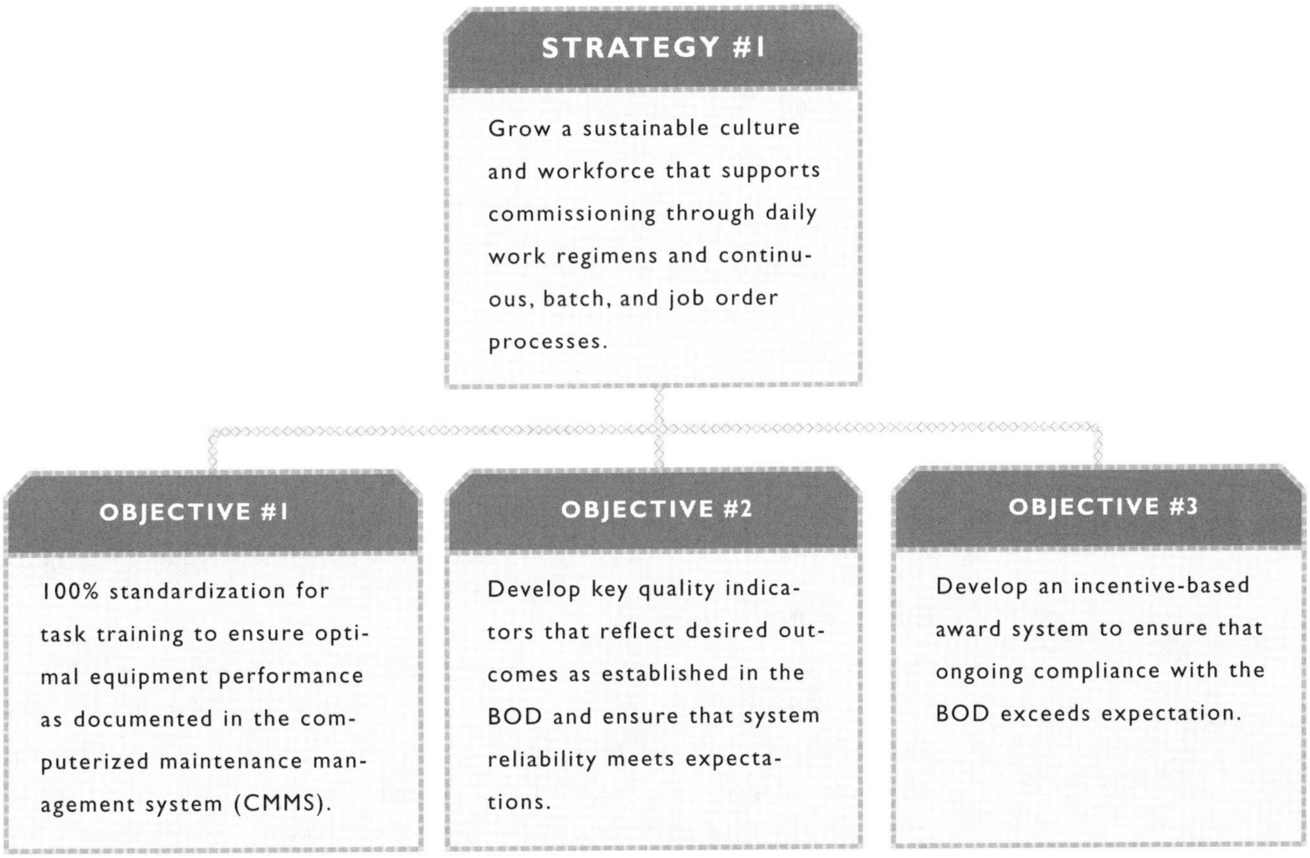

STRATEGY #1

Grow a sustainable culture and workforce that supports commissioning through daily work regimens and continuous, batch, and job order processes.

OBJECTIVE #1

100% standardization for task training to ensure optimal equipment performance as documented in the computerized maintenance management system (CMMS).

OBJECTIVE #2

Develop key quality indicators that reflect desired outcomes as established in the BOD and ensure that system reliability meets expectations.

OBJECTIVE #3

Develop an incentive-based award system to ensure that ongoing compliance with the BOD exceeds expectation.

As illustrated here, the four criteria of an MBO strategy set are:

- The strategy is realistic.
- Objectives are arranged in rank order.
- Objectives are stated quantitatively.
- Objectives are consistent.

Figure 1: Sample Management-by-Objectives Strategy

New Service Programs

The section on new service programs is where the real meat of the HFCx project argument is documented. Each strategy should be clearly defined, and tactics should be outlined to support each. Each strategy must answer these questions:

- What will be done?
- When will it be done?
- Who will do it?
- How much will it cost?
- How will progress be measured?
- How will effectiveness be measured?

Many health care business professionals will read the executive summary, then jump straight to the new service program section and the financial projections to understand the cost. This approach will give them a quick look at the project's purpose (briefed in the executive summary), an understanding of what the initiative will deliver in the physical world (tangible value derived as outlined in the new service program section), and a quick cost analysis. The new service programs section should properly document and support the HFCx initiative; do not take shortcuts when developing this section as the information in it will be the primary source the C-suite will use to evaluate the customer's derived outcomes and their willingness to fund the project.

Financial Projections

Cash is a scarce resource for most businesses, which makes the financial projections section a critical component of a great business plan.

Cash is a scarce resource for most businesses, which makes the financial projections section a critical component of a great business plan. Here, solid accounting practices and procedures are expected, and strong mathematical competence and scientific support are required to outpace other projects competing for the same resources. The best campaigns include analysis of the net present value (NPV) of a project, discounting future cash flows to present value to help health care business executives evaluate which project has the best internal rate of return (IRR).

The health care business executive's first priority is always to advance the core missions of the institution. These include patient care, education, and research, which will always garner a larger piece of the resource pie. However, the significant annual savings, reduced simple payback periods, and high returns on investment provided by many HFCx projects make a good impression. The best argument to support a great HFCx project proposal is the money that can be saved from the expense side of the balance sheet, dollar for dollar, which can then be invested in growing the primary missions of the institution—expanding patient care initiatives, improving research, and expanding education. In this context, the financial projections provide the C-suite with opportunities to support the greater good, improving the project's competitiveness and likelihood for funding.

Quality Controls

The final section of the business plan describes quality controls. Every project should be developed to ensure its success, but occasionally a project seems doomed from the beginning. Resistance may come from within, from outside the institution, and once in awhile from individuals who must change to support the initiative. Whatever the cause, sometimes a HFCx project is just not right for the institution and will not provide the desired outcomes. However, instituting some quality controls can help keep a project on track.

The business plan should include specific measures of success that were identified during the development phase. These metrics should be key quality indicators that can be monitored to determine progress as the project is delivered. Protocols should be included in the quality controls section that empower the project manager and health care facility executive to stop operations that are not contributing to the productive good of the enterprise. It is better to pull the plug after a $50,000 investment than to expend the full project cost of $250,000 and still not have a successful outcome.

In Sum

A business plan should be developed for every HFCx project regardless of its size. Smaller projects are easily documented, and the resources used to mount a successful campaign to fund the project with commissioning are only incrementally higher than what is required to present a project that has little opportunity for success. For larger projects, commissioning will ensure the project delivers the most cost-effective use of resources, meets the owner's project requirements, and prepares the operations and maintenance staff to maintain operational sustainability over the life cycle of the facility. Including a carefully prepared business plan with a request for scarce resources is always a good idea. Such a document can present the business case for health facility commissioning in your facility and help C-level reviewers understand its value.

A business plan should be developed for every HFCx project regardless of its size.

LEED® CERTIFICATION AND COMMISSIONING

Due to a number of factors—including the current health care business environment, diminishing fossil fuel supplies, escalating and volatile energy costs, global warming concerns, and a fragile electricity transmission grid—a growing percentage of the population now supports sustainable design and construction initiatives, which focus on stewardship of natural and fiscal resources. Many in the health care industry believe that a societal "tipping point" has been reached regarding the importance of green initiatives, and health care facilities often elect to employ sustainable design and construction practices on their projects. Such decisions are typically driven by environmental consciousness, stewardship, and energy conservation goals. In some cases, industry leaders believe that a visible demonstration of sustainable design and construction practices will yield an increase in philanthropic support of the health care facility.

A widely recognized indication of sustainable design and construction practices is LEED certification. LEED is an acronym for Leadership in Energy and Environmental Design, a sustainability rating system for buildings developed and promoted by the U.S. Green Building Council (USGBC). In recognition of the environmental benefits of commissioning, a minimum level of commissioning activity—referred to as "fundamental commissioning" of building energy systems—is a prerequisite for LEED certification. The minimum requirements of fundamental commissioning are as follows:

- The project team designates a HFCxA with documented commissioning experience in at least two projects. The HFCxA may be an independent third party, employee or consultant of the owner, employee of a company that is a member of the design team, or employee of the contractor or construction manager. However, the HFCxA cannot be directly involved with project design, construction, or construction management except for projects smaller than 50,000 square feet, when it is acceptable for a qualified person on the design or construction team to take on this responsibility. In any case, the HFCxA must report directly to the owner.

- The HFCxA reviews the owner's project requirements and the basis of design for clarity and completeness. The owner and the design team, respectively, update these documents as necessary.

- The project team includes commissioning requirements in the construction documents.

- The project team develops and implements a commissioning plan.

- The HFCxA verifies the installation and functional performance of the commissioned systems.

- The HFCxA documents the commissioning methodology and results in a written report.

At minimum, these energy-related components and systems must be commissioned during fundamental commissioning: HVAC equipment and systems and associated controls, alternative and renewable energy technologies, domestic hot water systems, and lighting and daylighting controls.

Additional LEED points can be earned by engaging in "enhanced commissioning," which requires the following in addition to the requirements of fundamental commissioning listed above:

- The HFCxA cannot be an employee of a company that is a member of the design team or an employee or consultant of the contractor or construction manager. The HFCxA may be contracted through the design firm.
- The HFCxA reviews the construction documents (approximately halfway through their production, followed by a "back-check" when the CDs are complete)
- The HFCxA reviews the submittal documents for the commissioned equipment for compliance with the OPR and BOD.
- The HFCxA creates a system manual.
- The HFCxA verifies that requirements for training are completed.
- The HFCxA is engaged to conduct a postoccupancy review.

It should be noted that a LEED® rating by itself does not ensure superior energy efficiency. A 2008 USGBC study of 121 new buildings certified through 2006, reported in *The New York Times* on August 31, 2009, found that 53 percent of the buildings would not qualify for the EPA Energy Star label and, perhaps even more alarmingly, 15 percent scored below 30 in the Energy Star program, indicating they are less efficient than 70 percent of comparable buildings. These statistics demonstrate that LEED certification and its fundamental commissioning prerequisite are not sufficient to ensure delivery of a high-performance building. Additional steps, including measurement and verification of actual building performance and ongoing commissioning, are required.

GLOSSARY

A comprehensive understanding of the commissioning process begins with the establishment of its own unique glossary of terms.

Acceptance phase: The phase of construction after start-up and initial check-out when functional performance tests, operations and maintenance documentation review, and operator training activities occur.

Approval: Acceptance that a piece of equipment or system has been properly installed and is functioning in tested modes according to the design intent.

Basis of design (BOD): Documentation of the systems, components, and methods used to meet the owner's project requirements. The BOD also documents the assumptions, alternatives, analysis, and thought processes used to establish the proposed design.

Building information modeling (BIM): Building information modeling is the process of generating and managing building data during its life cycle. Building information modeling uses three-dimensional, real-time, dynamic building modeling software to increase productivity in building planning, design, construction, maintenance, and operation. The process produces the building information model, which encompasses building geometry, spatial relationships, geographic information, and quantities and properties of building components.

Certificate of readiness: Documentation from the responsible party stating that each equipment/system is completely installed, functional, started up and all work has been completed prior to when functional testing is scheduled.

Commissioning: Process designed to ensure building systems perform in accordance with the design intent, the design intent is consistent with the owner's project requirements, and operations and maintenance staff are adequately prepared to operate and maintain the facility. Adequate preparation of the operations and maintenance staff includes training, documentation (record drawings, as-built drawings, etc.) and other resources (tools, gauges, thermometers, etc.).

Commissioning plan: Comprehensive plan that establishes the scope, structure, and schedule of the commissioning activities.

Commissioning team: All parties responsible for implementing the commissioning plan. The commissioning team may include the owner (C-level, facility manager, O&M staff), HFCxA, design team, and contractor.

Contract documents: Documents that establish the obligations of the design team, HFCxA, contractor, and other parties involved in a specific project. These include, but are not limited to, general conditions, specifications, change orders, and drawings. Typically, "contract documents" refers to the project drawings and specifications.

Contractor: Party responsible for constructing the project. Typically refers to the construction manager, general contractor, or subcontractors.

Control system: System and components associated with the control and operation of the building's mechanical and electrical systems. The control system typically includes networks, workstations, panels, controllers, and field devices such as sensors, valves, dampers, etc. The workstations, networks, and controllers are commonly referred to as the energy management system (EMS), building automation system (BAS), or utility monitoring and control system (UMCS).

Deferred functional tests: Functional tests performed after substantial completion due to partial occupancy, equipment, seasonal requirements, design or other site conditions that prevent the test from being performed during the construction phase of the project. Deferred functional tests are also referred as seasonal performance tests.

Deficiency: Condition of a component, piece of equipment, or system that is not compliant with the contract documents (i.e., does not perform properly or does not comply with design intent).

Design team: The architect, engineer, and other consultants responsible for development of the contract documens. The key design team players relevant to the commissioning process include the architect, electrical engineer, and mechanical engineer.

Energy Star: A joint program of the U.S. Environmental Protection Agency (EPA) and the U.S. Department of Energy designed to assist businesses and individuals in protecting the environment through superior energy efficiency. EPA's ENERGY STAR partnership offers a proven energy management strategy that helps in measuring current energy performance, setting goals, and tracking savings and rewards improvements.

Functional performance test (FPT): Test of dynamic function and operation that is conducted for components, equipment, systems, and integrated systems. Systems are tested under various modes (e.g., design loads, part loads, component failures, unoccupied periods, varying outside air temperatures, life safety conditions, power failure, etc.). Systems are run through all specified operational sequences. Components are verified to be responding in accordance with the contract documents. Functional performance tests are executed after pre-functional checklists, equipment start-ups, and contractor testing, adjusting, and balancing (TAB) are complete.

Functional performance test procedures: Commissioning protocols and detailed test procedures and instructions that fully describe the system configuration and steps required to determine if a system is performing and functioning properly. These procedures are used to perform and document functional performance tests.

Health facility commissioning (HFCx): A process intended to ensure that building systems are installed and perform in accordance with the design intent, that the design intent is consistent with the owner's project requirements, and that operations and maintenance staff are adequately prepared to operate and maintain the completed facility.

Health facility commissioning authority (HFCxA): Individual responsible for managing, coordinating, executing, and documenting the commissioning activities.

MEP equipment or systems: Mechanical/electrical/plumbing equipment or systems.

Monitoring: Recording of parameters (flow, current, status, pressure, temperature, humidity, etc.) of equipment operation using data loggers or trending capabilities of control systems.

Operation and maintenance (O&M) manuals: Documentation prepared by the construction team and vendors for use by O&M personnel in maintaining and operating the equipment and systems provided during the construction process. At minimum, these manuals generally include the following data for all commissioned equipment:

1. Name, address, and phone number of the installing contractor, subcontractors, vendors, and service organizations
2. Approved submittal data
3. Project- and site-specific operations and maintenance instructions, including model numbers and features that are clearly marked
4. Instructions for installation, maintenance, replacement, start-up, special maintenance, and replacement sources
5. A parts list
6. A list of special tools
7. Performance data
8. Warranty information

Overridden input: Temporarily changing an actual sensor value in a control system to determine and assess the response of the system (e.g., changing the outside air temperature value from 52 deg. F to 72 deg. F to verify economizer operation). *See also* "Simulated signal."

Overridden output: Writing over the programmed output in a control system to determine and assess the response of the system (e.g., opening an air terminal damper to verify proper reset of the static pressure set point). *See also* "Simulated signal."

Owner's project requirements (OPR): For a commissioning project, documentation that defines the functional requirements of a facility and the expectations of the owner as they relate to the systems to be commissioned. At a minimum, the OPR should establish the facility purpose, expected life, expected project cost, energy efficiency and sustainability goals, outdoor design conditions, and indoor environmental conditions.

Pre-functional checklist (PFC): A list of static inspections and elementary component tests that verify proper installation of equipment (e.g., installation and arrangement of associated services such as ductwork, piping, hydronic specialties, sensor locations, dampers, belt tension, oil levels, labels affixed, gauges in place, sensors calibrated, etc.).

Project manual: A document developed by the design team that establishes the general conditions of the contract for construction and the specifications.

Project team: All parties that have an interest in the project outcome, including the owner (C-level, facility manager, and O&M staff), program manager (if applicable), HFCxA, design team, and contractor.

Record drawings: A set of drawings revised by the contractor upon completion of a project to show as-built conditions. These drawings reflect all changes made in the specifications and working drawings during the construction process and show the exact dimensions, geometry, and location of all elements of the work completed under the contract.

Retrocommissioning: A systematic process that identifies low cost operational and maintenance improvements in an existing building that was not previously commissioned.

Seasonal performance tests: Functional performance tests deferred until ambient conditions reflect seasonal design conditions.

Shop drawings: Drawings created by a contractor, subcontractor, vendor, manufacturer, or other entity to illustrate construction, materials, dimensions, installation, and other information pertinent to the incorporation of an element or item into the construction.

Simulated condition: A condition created for testing a component or system (e.g., applying heat to a space temperature sensor to monitor the response of a VAV box).

Simulated signal: A signal generated by disconnecting a sensor and using a signal generator to send amperage, resistance, or pressure to a transducer and/or DDC system for the purpose of simulating value to the control system.

Specifications: Construction specifications in the contract documents.

Start-up: Initial testing and operation of systems or equipment. Start-up activities are completed prior to functional testing.

Subcontractor: Trade contractors contracted to the general contractor (GC) or construction manager (CM) who provide and install building components and systems.

Submittal documents: Drawings, data, samples, and so on that are submitted for review, evaluation, and approval prior to their inclusion in a project.

Systems manual: A manual focused on operating systems. At a minimum, it should include the final version of the OPR and the BOD, system single-line drawings, as-built sequences of operation, control shop drawings, original control set points, operating instructions for integrated systems, recommended retesting schedules and blank test forms, and sensor and actuator recalibration schedules. One of the manual's most important functions is provision of a condensed troubleshooting guide for O&M personnel at the system level.

Test procedure: A step-by-step process that must be executed to fulfill test requirements.

Testing requirements: Testing modes, functions, etc., specified in the HFCx plan. (Testing requirements are not detailed test procedures.)

Testing, adjusting, and balancing (TAB): A process by which the contractor tests, adjusts, and balances the air and hydronic systems. The contractor completes the TAB work prior to functional performance testing.

Trending: Monitoring the performance of commissioned systems over a defined period of time using the building control system.

Vendor: Supplier of equipment.

Warranty period: A period of time specified in the contract documents in which defects in workmanship, components, and equipment are corrected by the contractor at no cost to the owner.

PART 2

The Health Facility Commissioning Process

Predesign Phase

1.1 ESTABLISH THE COMMISSIONING SCOPE

The commissioning process begins with defining the commissioning scope by identifying the systems to be commissioned and the commissioning tasks to be performed for each system.

1.1.1 Systems to be Commissioned

The first step in establishing the scope for a commissioning project is to define the systems to be commissioned. A comprehensive commissioning scope for a health care facility should consider the items listed below.

(1) Building Envelope

  (a) Insulation

  (b) Glazing

  (c) Vapor barriers

  (d) All elements of the building exterior wall

  (e) Roof

  (f) Building pressure testing

(2) Life Safety

  (a) Fire-resistive ratings

  (b) Smoke barriers

  (c) Smoke-tight partitions

  (d) Stair pressurization system

  (e) Fire command center

(3) HVAC Systems

  (a) Air terminals

  (b) Induction units

  (c) Fan coil units

  (d) Unit heaters

  (e) Air handling units

  (f) Energy recovery units

  (g) Exhaust system

(h) Chilled water system

(i) Heating water system

(j) Steam system

(k) Humidifiers

(l) Fire and smoke dampers

(m) Special applications

- Operating rooms (anesthetizing locations)
- Airborne infection isolation (AII) rooms
- Protective environment (PE) rooms
- Data center
- Pharmacy
- Imaging

(4) Controls

(a) Workstations

(b) System graphics and dashboards

(c) Networks

(d) Controllers

(e) Sensors

(f) Actuators

(g) Meters

(5) Plumbing Systems

(a) Domestic cold water

- Meter
- Backflow preventers
- Booster pump
- Water softener

(b) Domestic hot water

- Water heater
- Recirculation system

(c) Sump pumps

(d) Natural gas

(e) Fuel oil

(f) Propane or synthetic natural gas

(g) Disinfection systems

(h) Rainwater harvesting

(i) Process cooling

(6) Medical Gas Systems

(a) Oxygen

(b) Bulk oxygen system

(c) Remote oxygen supply connection

(d) Nitrogen

(e) Nitrous oxide

(f) Medical vacuum

(g) Waste anesthesia gas disposal

(h) Instrument air

(i) Medical air

(j) Manifold rooms

(k) Master and area alarms

(l) Valves

- Source
- Future
- Riser
- Service
- Zone

(7) Electrical Systems

(a) Meter

(b) Primary transformers

(c) Main switchgear

(d) Panelboards

(e) Isolated power systems

(f) Power conditioners

(g) Power factor correction equipment

(h) Uninterruptible power supplies

(i) Step-down transformers

(j) Generators

(k) Paralleling switchgear

(l) Automatic transfer switches

(m) Lightning protection systems

(n) Grounding systems

(8) Fire Alarm System

(a) Workstations

(b) Controllers

(c) Sensing devices

(d) Interface with life safety systems

(e) Interface with fire protection system

(f) Interface with HVAC system

(g) Interface with elevators

(9) Information Technology

(a) Telephone

(b) Data

(c) Intercom

(d) Paging

(e) Doctor's dictation

(f) Telemetry

(g) Security

(h) Master clock

(i) Dedicated antenna

(j) Television

(k) Nurse call

(l) Infant abduction

(m) Wireless access points

(n) Cellular phone repeaters

(10) Fire Protection System

(a) Backflow preventer

(b) Fire pump/jockey pump

(c) Drains

(d) Tamper and flow switches

(e) Valves

(f) Fire department connections

(g) Standpipes

(h) Sprinkler heads

(i) Pre-action systems

(j) Clean agent systems

(11) Interior Lighting

(a) Occupancy sensors

(b) Controls

(12) Exterior Lighting

(a) Controls

(b) Illumination levels

(13) Refrigeration

(a) Food services refrigerators

(b) Food services freezers

(c) Clinical refrigerators and freezers

(d) Blood banks

(14) Vertical Transport

(a) Elevators

(b) Escalators

(c) Dumbwaiters

(15) Materials and Pharmaceutical Handling

(a) Pneumatic tube

(b) Linen and trash conveyance

(c) Electronic transportation vehicles (ETVs)

1.1.2 Factors Affecting the Commissioning Scope

(1) Reduced scope. The scope of a commissioning project may need to be reduced due to project size, schedule, or commissioning budget. A commissioning scope should be tailored to meet a project's needs based on the systems to be commissioned and tasks to be performed. Examples of areas that could be considered for reduced scope are as follows:

(a) On small projects or projects with limited budgets, commissioning may be limited to performing a plan review and documenting systems installation and function. In addition, the effort may be focused on major mechanical systems. The project scope should be developed to provide the greatest ROI for the facility.

(b) In some cases, the scope can be narrowed by testing only a representative sampling of selected systems. For example, terminal boxes in non-critical areas can be sampled at a 10 percent rate. If problems occur with the 10 percent sampling, then a larger percentage could be commissioned at the expense of the party who caused the failure. Sampling should be used to commission small, non-critical equipment such as terminal boxes, fan coil units, unit heaters, general purpose exhaust fans, CRACs, split systems, and so on.

(2) LEED certification. Projects with a LEED® certification goal must meet the minimum requirements for Energy and Atmosphere Prerequisite 1: Fundamental Commissioning of Building Energy Systems as defined in the current version of the LEED rating system. LEED projects may include additional scope for both systems and tasks such as those defined in Chapters 2 through 4 of the *Health Facility Commissioning Guidelines*.

1.2 SELECT THE COMMISSIONING PROJECT TEAM STRUCTURE

For the commissioning process, the health facility commissioning agent (HFCxA) serves as the owner's advocate and consultant. The HFCxA leads the commissioning team, which comprises representatives of the owner, design team, contractor, and subcontractors as well as the operations and maintenance (O&M) staff. As such, the HFCxA should be independent from ties to the project team that would represent a conflict of interest. The best way to accomplish this is for the HFCxA to be contracted directly to the owner. An independent third party will provide the most objective and unbiased services for the owner.

Members of the commissioning team such as the owner, contractor, or designer will possess knowledge of the systems involved in commissioning, but often they are heavily involved in issues related to delivering the project that are not related to commissioning. It is difficult for the design team to objectively review their design or analyze the effectiveness of specified control sequences. The construction team also has difficulty objectively assessing the installation of the equipment and systems they have installed and testing the functionality of these systems. As well, the urgency of the construction and occupancy schedules often compromise the constructor's objectivity and willingness to engage in detailed testing. These team members are generally not skilled at developing project-specific documents such as installation checklists or functional test procedures. In addition, they may not be skilled at executing the steps on the checklists, conducting the test procedures, or troubleshooting or diagnosing integration problems that often arise during functional testing.

With no responsibilities for the design and construction means and methods, a third-party HFCxA can focus on executing the tasks defined by the commissioning scope. Also, a third-party professional brings objectivity, commissioning experience, and team-building experience to the focused effort needed to effectively lead and coordinate the commissioning team.

1.3 SELECT THE HEALTH FACILITY COMMISSIONING AUTHORITY (HFCxA)

1.3.1 Timing

The HFCxA should be selected and engaged at the very outset of a project. An early engagement of the agent facilitates timely HFCxA design reviews and allows input before the design team has expended extensive effort on a specific design.

1.3.2 Qualifications

Commissioning is a professional service, and any requirements regarding professional engineering services are left to the discretion of the owner. Commissioning services are delivered by a firm specializing in commissioning (the HFCxA), which will provide a commissioning team for the project. The HFCxA should be selected based on qualifications that include key personnel, references, and experience.

The skill sets needed by a HFCxA are defined by the owner's commissioning project requirements.

1.3.3 Selection Process

The traditional process for selection of the HFCxA involves the following steps: first, establishment of a selection committee; second, advertisement and request for qualifications (RFQ); and third, interviews. In some instances, a request for proposal (RFP) is issued before the interviews to solicit detailed pricing information from short-listed firms.

(1) The selection committee. The owner appoints a selection committee, which typically includes three to five individuals, including the facility manager, user group representatives, and administrative representatives.

(2) Request for qualifications. The selection committee typically initiates the HFCxA selection process by issuing a request for qualifications. In the private sector, an advertisement may be placed or the RFQ may be sent to a list of potential HFCxAs identified by the selection committee. For public projects, the process generally involves a newspaper advertisement soliciting responses to the RFQ. Whether for public or private projects, the advertisement typically provides a general description of the project along with the project schedule, scope of commissioning services being sought, minimum qualifications required of the HFCxA, information that should be included in a proposal, and deadline for receipt of the response. For those responding to an RFQ, the required submission data should include:

(a) General description of the commissioning firm

(b) Organizational chart for the project team being offered by the HFCxA organization, including resumes of the proposed team members

(c) List of similar projects completed by the HFCxA organization and project team

(d) Roles and responsibilities of the proposed project team on previous projects listed as references in the submission

(e) Sample work products, such as commissioning plans, installation checklists, plan reviews, test procedures, and so on. (These may be required to demonstrate technical expertise and the degree of detail the HFCxA would provide in project-specific documents.)

(f) Recommended commissioning approach for the defined scope and the specific project

(3) Short list of qualified bidders. Sometimes a final HFCxA choice is made based solely on a review of RFQ responses, but most often the initial response results in selection of a short list of HFCxA firms. The short-listed group is then interviewed by the selection committee.

(4) Interviews. Interviews with prospective HFCxA organizations should be face-to-face discussions with the personnel who would

execute the process, including the proposed project manager and senior commissioning providers in each area of expertise (mechanical, electrical, low voltage, building envelope, etc.). Sufficient time should be allowed for the project team to discuss its process as well as any specific topics the selection committee would like to address. Each interview should also allow time for questions and answers.

1.3.4 Making the Decision

The HFCxA selection process is most successful when the selection committee bases its choice on the provider's qualifications. Once the HFCxA has been selected, the selection committee and the HFCxA can negotiate fees to match the scope of services required. However, when circumstances require the selection to be based on proposed fee as well as qualifications, the HFCxA qualifications should be the over-riding factor. A more qualified HFCxA can yield significant cost savings in other aspects of the total cost, which will more than offset a relatively small difference in fee.

See Appendix A for a sample RFP for commissioning services.

1.4 NEGOTIATE THE HFCxA FEE AND CONTRACT

The HFCxA fee should be based on the scope of commissioning services and the size of the project. Differences among projects—such as the construction schedule, project phasing, types of systems used, size of the equipment used, and so on—make it difficult to offer a precise estimating tool for commissioning services. However, there are some rules of thumb that can be used. Fees for small projects will be more expensive per square foot or as a percentage of construction cost than fees for larger projects. The same can be said for project scopes, which can vary from simple to complex. Commissioning fees for the ASHE HFCx process should typically be in the range of 0.50 percent of the total construction cost for extremely large projects and up to 1.25 percent for small projects.

As a representative and advocate of the owner, the HFCxA must work directly for the owner without any type of intermediary. Further, a direct relationship between the owner and the HFCxA is absolutely essential to ensure complete objectivity. The agreement between the owner and the HFCxA should be fair to both parties and represent a fee based on the scope defined.

A sample contract for commissioning services is provided in Appendix B.

Design Phase

2.1 ORGANIZE AND ATTEND THE PREDESIGN CONFERENCE

The HFCxA should organize and attend a predesign conference at the beginning of the design phase. The conference should be attended—at least—by representatives of the owner, architect, engineer, and contractor (if engaged at this stage of the process). For the conference to be productive, it is essential that these representatives have the authority to make a decision on behalf of their organizations (including the owner). The predesign conference establishes the commissioning process for the project and the specific roles and responsibilities of each individual and firm involved. The HFCxA should prepare an agenda for the meeting and forward it to all parties well in advance of the conference.

The meeting should begin with discussions about the project goals, scope, team members, and delivery process. These discussions should address the project budget, schedule, and performance expectations. After all parties have been introduced to the project, the HFCxA should provide a detailed description of the anticipated commissioning process and define the specific roles and responsibilities of each individual and firm.

2.2 SET PROJECT ENERGY EFFICIENCY GOALS

The HFCxA should work with the owner, design team, and contractor to establish an aggressive yet attainable and fiscally responsible energy efficiency goal. This goal should be set using the EPA Energy Star Target Finder tool, which can be accessed from www.energystar.gov. The Target Finder provides weather normalized (based on zip code) energy efficiency goals for health care facilities and other types of commercial buildings.

The project team uses the Target Finder to determine site and source energy use and cost targets for a project at a specific location associated with a defined Energy Star rating, energy fuel mix, and energy unit prices. For new facilities, the recommended Energy Star target rating is 75 (the minimum required to earn the Energy Star label). For renovation and building addition projects, the recommended Energy Star target rating should be a reasonable increase from the current and baseline energy ratings for the existing facility. Figure 2-1 illustrates the percentile rating system used by the EPA Energy Star program.

1 to 100 Benchmark Scale

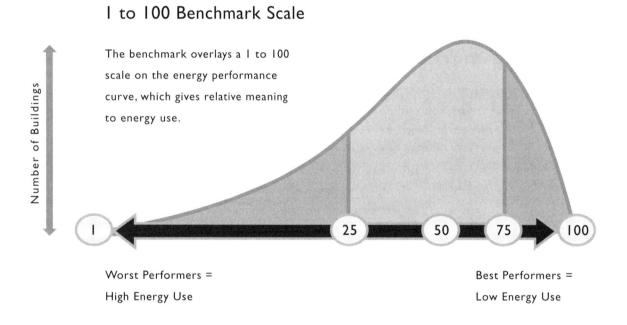

The benchmark overlays a 1 to 100 scale on the energy performance curve, which gives relative meaning to energy use.

Worst Performers =
High Energy Use

Best Performers =
Low Energy Use

Figure 2-1: EPA Benchmark Scale

After the site and source energy use and cost targets have been determined, the design team should develop predictions of energy use and cost using a building simulation program (commonly referred to as an "energy model"). If the predicted energy use and cost values are higher than the Energy Star targets, the HFCxA should work with the owner, design team, and contractor to identify and evaluate potential energy conservation measures. The evaluation should consider impacts on capital cost, schedule, energy efficiency, operating costs, and life cycle costs. Energy conservation measures found to be cost-effective (i.e., that generate returns higher than the facility's weighted cost of capital) should be incorporated into the final design. The identification, evaluation, and incorporation process should be repeated until the predicted energy use and cost associated with the final design are consistent with the Energy Star targets.

A facility designed to achieve an Energy Star rating of 75 or higher is eligible to receive the EPA's "Designed to Earn the Energy Star" designation.

2.3 FACILITATE DEVELOPMENT OF THE OWNER'S PROJECT REQUIREMENTS (OPR)

2.3.1 Timing and Content for the OPR

After the project team has been selected, the owner's expectations and requirements for the commissioned equipment and systems should be documented in writing. This document, typically referred to as the owner's project requirements (OPR), should be developed at project inception.

The OPR should detail the functional requirements for the building being designed as well as the expectations for its use and operation as they relate to the systems being commissioned. Included should be project goals, cost requirements, measurable performance criteria; owner-provided guidelines and standards; and the criteria that will be used to measure the success of the project.

The owner, design team, and HFCxA should work collaboratively to develop the OPR. Key stakeholders on the project team and the owner's staff must contribute to its development as well. This is readily accomplished by holding an OPR charrette—a working session for brainstorming—to gather input.

From the data gathered during the charrette, a draft of the OPR can be developed for final review and comment by the participants. The finalized OPR is published, but the document continues to be modified as the project progresses through the design and construction phases.

The OPR is a dynamic and living document that should be updated periodically throughout the planning, design, and construction process.

Refer to Appendix C for a sample OPR.

2.3.2 Key Elements of the OPR

(1) Background—A narrative description to provide context for the project. Define the primary purpose of the project, the program needs, flexibility in the project program, and future expansion requirements.

(2) Objectives—A complete list of the goals and objectives for the project, including first cost, change orders, life cycle cost, energy efficiency, infection rates, patient and visitor satisfaction scores, staffing requirements, maintenance costs, services, floor area, capacity for future growth, and schedule. (The energy efficiency goal should be consistent with the targeted Energy Star rating.)

(3) Functional program—A document developed by the owner and architect to establish the specific purpose and use of each space in the health care facility (e.g., dining rooms, patient rooms, operating rooms, office, kitchen, storage, etc.). The functional program should also include any specific requirements for design of each functional area, including security, safety, comfort requirements, energy consumption, maintainability, etc. Authorities having jurisdiction (AHJs) use the functional program to determine applicable codes and regulations.

(4) Life span, cost, and quality—Documentation of the owner's expectations for the life span of systems and components, the cost of construction, and the level of quality desired, and so on. Define the level of reliability expected from the equipment, the level of automation and flexibility desired from building systems, any desired technologies and preferred manufacturers, and so on.

(5) Performance criteria—Minimum acceptable performance benchmarks for various aspects of the facility. For example, a target Energy Star rating should be established, and facility performance should be linked to the ASHE E2C program.

(6) Maintenance requirements—A description of how the facility will be operated and by whom, along with the level of training needed for the O&M staff to understand the systems and staffing required to operate and maintain them. This should include specific aspects of the design that operations and maintenance (O&M) personnel will need to understand to facilitate system operation and maintenance (e.g., operating and maintenance dashboards and associated meters and sensors) and commissioning tools to be used to query the automatic temperature control system and other components. (The maintenance requirements will depend on both the level of knowledge of the current O&M staff and the expected complexity of the proposed systems, and any significant gap between the two must be addressed.)

2.4 FACILITATE DEVELOPMENT OF THE BASIS OF DESIGN FOR SYSTEMS TO BE COMMISSIONED

After the OPR is complete, the means and methods to be used to incorporate the owner's project requirements for the systems to be commissioned into the facility design should be documented in writing. This document is typically referred to as the basis of design (BOD) and is usually developed by the design team.

The BOD is a dynamic and living document that is periodically updated throughout the planning, design, and construction process.

Refer to Appendix D for a sample BOD.

2.4.1 BOD Content

The BOD should begin with descriptions of the building (including floor area and number of floors) and the building envelope (including roof, walls, glazing, vapor barriers, R values, etc.). The BOD should also identify the following:

(1) Applicable codes and standards

(2) Outdoor design conditions (e.g., geography, weather)

(3) Indoor design conditions (e.g., temperature, relative humidity, air changes, etc.)

(4) Expected building occupancy for all building uses (including nights, weekends, holidays, special events, etc.)

(5) Miscellaneous power loads for all building occupancies

(6) Illumination levels, controls, and power requirements for all building occupancies

(7) Other internal loads

(8) Ventilation requirements for all building occupancies

(9) Building infiltration and pressure requirements

(10) Anticipated maintenance management program

(11) Maintenance and service requirements for all commissioned systems

(12) Indoor air quality requirements

(13) Acoustics criteria for HVAC system

(14) Life safety criteria (fire protection, fire alarm, and smoke control)

(15) Sustainable design elements

(16) Energy conservation measures

2.5. REVIEW THE OPR AND BOD

The HFCxA reviews the OPR and BOD and verifies that they are comprehensive, specific to the project, and clearly understandable. The HFCxA also verifies that the OPR identifies all appropriate goals and objectives and that the designs, equipment, and systems identified in the BOD are responsive to the goals and objectives established by the OPR. The HFCxA also reviews the OPR and BOD with hospital O&M staff and documents their comments and concerns. The HFCxA prepares a written list of comments and forwards the list to the owner and the design team.

2.6 REVIEW THE SCHEMATIC DESIGN DOCUMENTS

2.6.1 Design Review Scope

The HFCxA reviews the documents produced by the design team. In other commissioning guidelines, the scope of the HFCxA design review is restricted to commissionability considerations only. The ASHE commissioning guidelines, on the other hand, require the HFCxA to review the design documents with a focus on commissionability, completeness, cost-effectiveness, coordination of trades, and energy efficiency.

The HFCxA design reviews should accomplish the following tasks:

- Verify that the design documents are complete and contain the information required for construction, maintenance, and operations.
- Suggest alternative designs that might yield a lower project cost without adversely affecting performance.
- Suggest alternative designs that might reduce energy costs, maintenance costs, and life cycle costs without unduly increasing the construction cost.

2.6.2 Schematic Design Review

In reviewing the schematic design documents, the HFCxA verifies that the documents are consistent with the OPR and BOD and that the proposed design conforms to best practice.

The HFCxA also reviews the schematic design documents with hospital O&M staff and documents their comments and concerns. The HFCxA prepares a written list of all comments and forwards it to the owner and the design team.

The HFCxA follows up with the design team to ensure written responses to the review comments are provided.

2.7 DEVELOP THE COMMISSIONING PLAN

2.7.1 Development of the Plan

The HFCxA develops a health facility commissioning (HFCx) plan for the commissioning team to follow. The plan is a comprehensive document that describes the commissioning process and how it will be executed. It includes project-specific pre-functional checklists and functional performance test procedures. The commissioning plan is distributed to the commissioning team for review and comment before it is finalized.

   The commissioning plan is a dynamic document that evolves as the design and construction progress continues.

2.7.2 Commissioning Plan Components

(1) Overview—A brief overview of the commissioning process that addresses the design, construction, acceptance, occupancy, operational, and warranty phases of commissioning.

(2) List of equipment and systems—A master equipment list that includes descriptions of the equipment and systems to be commissioned. Each piece of equipment on the list is associated with a system. As well, the part of the building served and related systems that interface with it are indicated for each system and piece of equipment. This information on this list will be used to schedule completion of systems and to track completion of the commissioning process.

(3) Team roles—A description of the roles of the commissioning team members, who traditionally include the owner, design professionals, contractors, and HFCxA. The design team defines the scope, the contractors complete the work and demonstrate its performance (under the direction of the commissioning authority) and the HFCxA develops procedures for demonstrating installation and operation based on the contract documents. The HFCxA will document completion in interim reports, review items that require follow-up, and document the final status of commissioned systems in the final commissioning report. The owner will operate and maintain the commissioned systems once the project is complete.

(4) Management and communication—A description of the management, communication, and reporting of the commissioning process.

(5) Deliverables—Expected work products of the commissioning process.

(6) Commissioning milestones—Key milestones of the commissioning process.

(7) Start-up—A matrix defining all start-up requirements of the construction documents. The commissioning specifications require the contractor to develop a start-up and initial systems checkout plan. That plan will be describe how the manufacturer's start-up process interfaces with the initial commissioning pre-functional testing procedures. It also describes how the sub-elements of a system must be completed and started functional testing of complete systems is conducted.

(8) Installation checklists—Pre-functional checklists (PFC) for each piece of equipment and system in the scope of commissioning work. The PFCs are created to document that installation of the equipment and systems is in accordance with the design requirements. These checklists, developed from the requirements of the plans and specifications, combine all installation requirements for a piece of equipment and break them down into categories. For example, the PFC for an air-conditioning unit will address the installation clearance, serviceability, coil piping arrangements, electrical connections, duct and plenum connections, insulation, labeling, filters, and control component rough-in all in one checklist. The checklists are created during the design phase and updated during construction to reflect modifications should they occur as a result of shop drawing reviews or scope revisions.

(9) Functional testing—Functional performance test (FPT) procedures for each piece of equipment and system that is to be commissioned. These procedures are created to establish the testing process and performance expectations for each piece of equipment, system, and integrated system developed from the contract document requirements. These procedures will describe how equipment and systems are to be tested to demonstrate they operate as the design intended. The tests will include temperature controls, safeties and alarms, air volume control, and operation on normal and emergency power as well as transfer of power, humidity control, normal and emergency power distribution, the fire alarm system and its interface with the HVAC system, the smoke evacuation system, elevators, the fire sprinkler system and fire pump, and so on. These test procedures are created during the design phase and updated during construction to reflect modifications should they occur as a result of shop drawing reviews or scope revisions.

(10) Training—A list of the training required in the contract scope. Where detailed training plans, scheduling, and coordination with the owner's needs and staff schedules are required, this information is included on the list.

(11) Operations and maintenance manuals—A list of the O&M documentation required per the contract scope. When required, this list will include the detailed format for these documents, specific submission requirements, availability for owner training, and so on.

(12) Opposed season testing and warranty reviews—A list of the opposed season and warranty items that are required, with a definition of the process for monitoring execution of these activities.

2.8 PREPARE THE COMMISSIONING SPECIFICATIONS

2.8.1 Preparation of the Specifications

The HFCxA prepares the commissioning specifications, which define the specific scope of work, roles and responsibilities, and requirements for each member of the commissioning team. The design team inserts the commissioning specifications into the project manual, as the construction team needs to see them to accurately price the cost of the work.

2.8.2 Commissioning Specifications Elements

At minimum, the commissioning specifications should address the following:

(1) Commissioning team involvement

(2) Contractor's responsibilities

(3) Submittals and submittal review procedures for HFCxA process/systems

(4) Operation and maintenance documentation/systems manual requirements

(5) Number of project meetings related to commissioning and which commissioning team members are obligated to participate

(6) Construction verification procedures

(7) Start-up plan development and implementation

(8) Functional performance test procedures

(9) Acceptance and closeout procedures

(10) Training requirements, including development of a training plan

(11) Warranty review site visit

2.9 REVIEW THE DESIGN DEVELOPMENT DOCUMENTS

The HFCxA reviews the design development documents prepared by the design team. Objectives for this review include:

- Verify consistency with the BOD and OPR.

- Verify that HFCxA and owner comments from the schematic design review have been addressed.

- Assess whether the space allocation, equipment layouts, maintainability, coordination of systems, and general equipment sizing (capacities) in the documents are adequate to meet the owner's needs.

- Confirm that redundancy and future capacity issues have been addressed on the drawings.

- Verify that the design includes the features needed to execute the HFCx plan.

The HFCxA also reviews the design development documents with hospital O&M staff and documents their comments and concerns. The HFCxA prepares a written list of comments and forwards the list to the owner and the design team.

The HFCxA follows up with the design team to ensure that written responses to the review comments are provided.

2.10 REVIEW THE HVAC CONTROL SYSTEM SEQUENCES OF OPERATION

Design engineers write HVAC equipment sequences of operation in standard text-based format. These sequences typically describe the control process in general terms without much detail. Highly trained programmers employed by the control system supplier then write the actual system control programs using a process control language.

Many buildings fail to perform in accordance with expectations because the actual control system programming is not consistent with the intended equipment sequences of operation. This disparity has several causes. First, the text format sequence of operation written by the design engineer may not be sufficiently detailed. For example, a design engineer might write the following air-handling unit sequence of operation:

When the economizer mode is enabled, modulate the preheat control valve, mixed air dampers, and chilled water control valve as required to maintain the supply air temperature at set point.

The control system programmer might respond to this sequence by writing separate proportional–integral (PI) loop statements for each controlled device. This approach would likely yield proper control of the supply air temperature, but unfortunately, the individual loop statements could overlap and cause simultaneous heating and cooling. A situation of this type is particularly troublesome as the energy waste associated with it might go undetected indefinitely because the supply air temperature falls within a normal range and the building occupants do not complain. To ensure proper control as well as energy efficiency, the design engineer should revise the sequence as indicated below:

> When the economizer mode is enabled, modulate the preheat control valve, mixed air dampers, and chilled water control valve *in sequence* as required to maintain the supply air temperature at set point *using a single proportional-integral loop statement and separate table statements for each controlled device.*

To ensure that building energy efficiency targets are met, the design engineer must prepare detailed sequences of operation that address all aspects of intended performance, including adjustable set points, non-adjustable set points, weekly schedules, alarms, warnings, trends, tuning, and energy-efficient processes. The HFCxA should carefully review these sequences and make certain they contain adequate detail and incorporate energy-efficient processes (e.g., static pressure set point reset, supply air temperature set point reset, occupancy sensors, unoccupied/occupied air change rates, weekly scheduling with optimal start/stop, etc.).

2.11 REVIEW THE CONSTRUCTION DOCUMENTS

2.11.1 Review Process

The HFCxA reviews the construction documents prepared by the design team.

The HFCxA also reviews the construction documents with hospital O&M staff and documents their comments and concerns. The HFCxA prepares a written list of comments and forwards the list to the owner and the design team.

The HFCxA follows up with the design team to ensure written responses to the review comments are provided.

2.11.2 Objectives

(1) Verify consistency with the BOD and OPR.

(2) Verify that the comments from the HFCxA and owner submitted after the design development review have been addressed.

(3) Review major equipment capacity information provided against general experience for similar facilities.

(4) Review sequences of operation for clarity, completeness, and energy efficiency.

(5) Assess accessibility to valves, gauges, thermometers, dampers, control components, etc.

(6) Spot-check above-ceiling clearances to ensure adequate space is provided for access/maintenance of all above-ceiling MEP equipment (valves, air terminal units, dampers, etc.).

(7) Assess adequacy for operations and maintenance of quantity and location of sensors, flow-measuring stations, and so on. Even consider features beyond those required to control the system.

(8) Do a spot-check comparison of the design development review comments and the construction documents to ensure the comments have been picked up and that adequate space allocation, equipment layouts, maintainability, and coordination of systems are provided

(9) Check for sufficient isolation valves, dampers, interlocks, and piping so that conditions can be simulated for overrides, failures, etc.

(10) Check the documents for coordination between disciplines for requirements for system integration.

2.12 UPDATE THE COMMISSIONING PLAN AND COMMISSIONING SPECIFICATIONS

As the construction documents near completion, the HFCxA updates the commissioning plan and commissioning specifications. The updated documents should be detailed and project-specific. The HFCxA also develops the final pre-functional checklists and functional performance tests and attaches them to the commissioning plan.

These updated documents are issued with the final construction documents.

2.13 FACILITATE DEVELOPMENT OF THE UTILITY MANAGEMENT PLAN

2.13.1 Purpose of the UMP

The Joint Commission and similar organizations accredit many health care facilities. Accreditation provides "deemed status," whereby the facility is deemed to be compliant with the Centers for Medicare and Medicaid Services (CMS) Conditions of Participation (COP). Compliance is required for a health care facility to receive reimbursement from the Medicare and Medicaid programs. One requirement in the Joint Commission's *2010 Comprehensive Accreditation Manual for Hospitals* is development of a comprehensive utility management plan (UMP).

Even if the UMP is not required for a specific facility, it is an industry-accepted best practice and should be developed. Health care facility mainte-nance personnel use the UMP to manage utilities during an emergency (Joint Commission Emergency Management Standard EM.02.02.09) and manage risks associated with utility systems (Joint Commission Environment of Care Standard EC.02.05.01).

2.13.2 Process for Development

Because the design and construction of utility systems has a significant effect on the policies and procedures established in the UMP, the HFCxA should work with the facility manager, design team, and contractor to facilitate devel-opment of the plan prior to completion of the final design. After the project team has developed the UMP, the HFCxA submits it to the facility manager.

2.13.3 UMP Components

(1) Written inventories of the operating components of utility systems considered critical to patient care based on risks of infection and occupant needs, including these:

   (a) Chilled water systems

   (b) Heating water systems

   (c) Domestic cold water systems

   (d) Sanitary sewer systems

   (e) Natural gas systems

   (f) Fuel oil systems

   (g) Fire alarm systems

   (h) Medical vacuum systems

   (i) Medical air systems

   (j) Medical gas systems

   (k) Steam systems

   (l) Fire protection systems

   (m) Normal power systems

   (n) Essential power systems

   (o) Nurse call systems

(p) HVAC systems

(q) Pneumatic tube systems

(r) Vertical transportation systems

(2) Written descriptions of the inspection, testing, and maintenance activities for operating components of critical utility systems

(3) Detailed diagrams of utility distribution systems

(4) Written procedures for responding to utility system disruptions

(5) Written procedures for shutting off malfunctioning utility systems and notifying staff in affected areas

(6) Written procedures for obtaining emergency repair services

(7) Written identification of alternative means of providing electricity, water, and fuel

(8) Written identification of alternative means for providing medical air, medical vacuum, oxygen, nitrous oxide, nitrogen, and other medical gases

(9) Written identification of alternative means of providing other critical utilities, such as vertical transport, steam for sterilization, heating, cooling, and ventilation

(10) Written procedures for responding to events that curtail or disrupt utility service to the health care facility for up to 96 hours

2.14 ATTEND THE PRE-BIDDING CONFERENCE

The HFCxA attends the pre-bidding conference(s) and answers questions regarding commissioning.

Construction Phase

3.1 CONDUCT THE COMMISSIONING CONFERENCE

After the bidding/pricing of the construction documents is complete and before construction starts, the HFCxA organizes and attends the commissioning conference. The commissioning conference is a meeting of the HFCxA, owner, contractor, subcontractors, and design team. Its purpose is to review the commissioning plan and commissioning specifications to make certain that all parties fully understand the commissioning process and their assigned roles and responsibilities. The commissioning conference should specifically address the process for submittal review and approval that is established in the project manual and commissioning specifications.

3.2 DEVELOP AND MAINTAIN THE ISSUES LOG

During the course of design and construction, the HFCxA maintains a log of all identified issues and concerns. The log includes a definition of each issue, the date it was identified, a proposed corrective plan, the party responsible, the date of anticipated resolution, and its current status. At the completion of the project, the issues log documentation provides a comprehensive list of all commissioning-related issues and their resolution.

3.3 REVIEW SUBMITTAL DATA AND SHOP DRAWINGS

The HFCxA reviews all submittal documents related to the commissioned systems. The purpose of these reviews is to ensure conformance with the commissioning plan, commissioning specifications, and OPR. The HFCxA also reviews these documents with operations and maintenance (O&M) personnel and forwards comments and concerns in writing to the design team and the owner. The design team reviews these and considers incorporating the items into the design team's formal review process. The project team then discusses and resolves any HFCxA and O&M personnel comments and concerns that the design team does not incorporate into its formal review.

3.4 REVIEW OPERATIONS & MAINTENANCE MANUALS

Contractors must submit O&M manuals for approval as soon as possible after their shop drawings have been approved. The HFCxA then reviews the manuals to ensure proper content and format. Frequently these documents are not suitable for use by the maintenance staff. Common problems include lack of organization, poor editing (not specific to the project), and incomplete content. The HFCxA prepares a written list of deficiencies in the manuals and sends a copy to the owner, contractor, and design team. The HFCxA review ensures the manuals contain the information and guidance required for effective operation and maintenance of the commissioned systems and equipment.

The manuals should be available to operations personnel prior to and during training. As reference materials for the operation of systems, these documents are essential to the training process.

Requirements for the manuals should be specified by the design team with input from the facility O&M staff. The specification should define the level of detail required, the document organization, the delivery process, and the timing for completion of the manuals (after approval of shop drawings and before owner training).

The HFCxA reviews the manuals and documents whether:

- Manuals are provided for all equipment to be commissioned.
- Manuals are organized as specified. (When submitted as paper copies rather than electronically, manuals are properly bound and labeled.)
- Manuals include specified project-specific data only, such as:
  — Name, address, and phone number of the installing contractor and vendor
  — Approved submittal data
  — Project- and site-specific operations and maintenance instructions, including model numbers and features that are clearly marked
  — Instructions for installation, maintenance, replacement, start-up, special maintenance, and replacement sources
  — A parts list
  — A list of special tools
  — Performance data
  — Warranty information

The HFCxA also reviews the manuals with O&M personnel and forwards comments and concerns in writing to the design team and owner. The design team then reviews the HFCxA comments and concerns and considers incorporating these items into the design team formal review process. The project team then discusses and resolves any HFCxA and O&M personnel comments and concerns the design team has not incorporated into its formal review.

3.5 CONDUCT COMMISSIONING MEETINGS

During the course of construction, the HFCxA conducts commissioning meetings. Held as needed to facilitate commissioning activities, these should be organized, brief, and meaningful for all parties. It is helpful to hold "milestone meetings" at the beginning of each phase of commissioning, including the following:

- Shop drawing submission
- Equipment installation
- Pre-functional checklists
- Equipment start-up
- Functional performance testing
- Submission of operating and maintenance manuals
- Owner training
- Seasonal testing

3.6 ATTEND SELECTED PROJECT MEETINGS

The HFCxA reviews the minutes of the regular project meetings and attends selected project meetings as needed to resolve issues and concerns and coordinate the commissioning process.

3.7 LEAD O&M STAFF CONSTRUCTION SITE TOURS

The HFCxA leads facility O&M personnel on regular tours of the construction site, discussing the equipment, systems, OPR, BOD, scheduled maintenance requirements, sequences of operation, and so on. The HFCxA maintains a list of their comments and concerns and works with the contractor and design team to respond to these using the standard issues log format. The HFCxA encourages the maintenance staff to become stakeholders in a positive construction outcome.

3.8 COMPLETE PRE-FUNCTIONAL CHECKLISTS AND INSPECTIONS

Equipment installations are reviewed to verify compliance with the construction documents. These reviews are documented using pre-functional checklists (PFCs) developed by the HFCxA or the owner from information on the design drawings, shop drawings, etc. The PFCs are developed and executed in phases (e.g., equipment installation, piping rough-in, electrical rough-in, controls rough-in, feeder and load side termination for electrical systems, etc.) as the work progresses. Any deficiencies noted during the installation phases are discussed with the commissioning team during site visits, documented in the master issues log, and included in site visit reports. Resolution of deficiencies is documented on subsequent site visits. All elements of equipment and system installation and all PFCs must be complete prior to functional testing.

If it is not feasible for the HFCxA or the owner to execute the PFCs, this task can be carried out by other members of the commissioning team, including the contractor or the design team. However, when pre-functional checklists and inspections are executed by the contractor or design team, the HFCxA should review a randomly selected representative sample of completed PFCs throughout the construction process to ensure consistency and quality.

3.9 REVIEW HVAC CONTROL SYSTEM PROGRAMMING

One cause of the frequent disparity between the text format sequence and the actual control program is a language barrier between the design engineer and the control system programmer. The design engineer may not be familiar with the actual process control language used by the automatic temperature control system, and the control system programmer may not be familiar with HVAC systems and equipment.

To bridge this communication gap, the HFCxA must review the actual control system programming and make certain it conforms to the design intent. The HFCxA should review the programs before implementation and again after implementation to ensure proper performance.

3.10 WITNESS EQUIPMENT AND SYSTEMS START-UP

The HFCxA reviews equipment start-up procedures, witnesses the start-up of critical systems, and reviews the completed start-up documentation.

3.11 REVIEW TAB REPORT

The HFCxA reviews the testing, adjusting, and balancing (TAB) report prepared by the contractor and prepares a written response to it, which is distributed to the owner, contractor, and design team. The HFCxA should also spot-check a representative sample of airflow and water flow readings as documented in the TAB report. The duration of the sampling should be definable (e.g., two eight-hour days).

3.12 WITNESS FUNCTIONAL PERFORMANCE TESTS

The HFCxA directs comprehensive equipment and system testing. These functional performance tests are conducted after all other elements of equipment and system installation—including pre-functional inspections and checklists, equipment start-up, and contractor testing—have been completed. The purpose of the functional performance tests is to ensure the systems perform in accordance with the design intent.

The functional performance tests assess the performance of the commissioned systems under design, part load, and emergency conditions. The tests are conducted by proceeding from simple system to complex system to integrated systems testing. The HFCxA asks operations and maintenance personnel to attend and witness the functional performance tests as the testing process provides great insight into the intended system operation and function.

3.13 FACILITATE PRESSURE TESTING

3.13.1 Code Requirements

Current codes require controlled pressure relationships between critical health care spaces such as operating rooms, procedure rooms, airborne infection isolation (AII) rooms, and protective environment (PE) rooms and adjacent spaces. Differences between supply and return/exhaust airflow rates, frequently referred to as offsets, create these pressure relationships. The amount of offset required to create a specific pressure relationship is a function of the effective room leakage area. Figure 2-2 illustrates the relationship between effective room leakage area, offset, and pressure difference.

As indicated in Figure 2-2, the airflow offset required to create a 0.01 in. w.g. (inches water gauge) pressure difference with an effective room leakage area of 1.50 square feet is 400 CFM (cubic feet per minute). The actual amount of effective room leakage area is a function of building and room construction and is difficult to predict in advance. Since an increase in effective

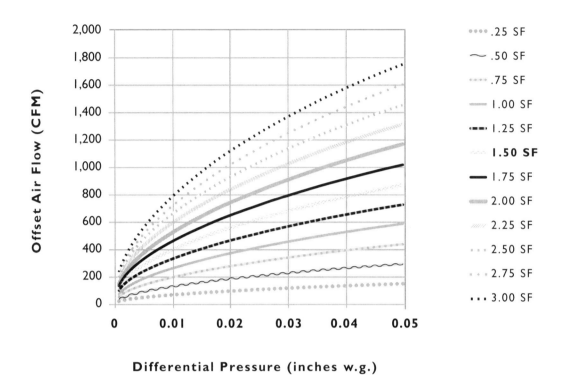

Figure 2-2: Relationship between Airflow Offsets, Differential Pressure, and Effective Leakage Area

leakage area increases the required offset, which in turn increases system airflow and fan energy consumption, a higher than expected effective leakage area adversely affects energy costs.

3.13.2 Steps for Positive Pressure Rooms

To ensure proper system operation and limit energy costs, the commissioning process should include pressure testing of all areas requiring controlled pressure relationships (e.g., AII and PE rooms). The recommended pressure testing process for positive pressure rooms includes these steps:

(1) Close all doors to the room.

(2) Seal off exhaust/return air grilles.

(3) Increase the supply air terminal airflow set point until the room differential pressure is equal to the desired value.

(4) Record the supply airflow and the room differential pressure.

(5) Determine the amount of effective leakage area using the relationship shown in Figure 2-2.

(6) If the amount of effective leakage area is higher than anticipated, the contractor should identify and seal leaks.

(7) The testing and sealing process is then repeated until the effective leakage area is acceptable.

3.13.3 Steps for Testing Negative Pressure Rooms

The recommended pressure testing process for negative pressure rooms includes these steps:

(1) Close all doors to the room.

(2) Close the supply air terminal damper.

(3) Seal off the supply air diffusers.

(4) Increase the exhaust air terminal airflow set point until the room differential pressure is equal to the desired value.

(5) Record the exhaust airflow and the room differential pressure.

(6) Determine the amount of effective leakage area using Figure 2-2.

(7) If the amount of effective leakage area is higher than anticipated, the contractor should identify and seal leaks.

(8) The testing and sealing process is then repeated until the effective leakage area is acceptable.

3.13.4 Steps for Testing the Building Envelope

Controlling building pressure is also critical to efficient and comfortable building operation. The building pressure relative to the outdoors at the main entry should be very close to neutral. The amount of outside air in excess of the building exhaust required to create an appropriate building pressure depends on the integrity of the building envelope. To ensure the building envelope is properly sealed, the commissioning process should include building pressure testing.

The recommended pressure testing process for the building envelope includes these steps:

(1) Close all doors and openings to the building.

(2) Verify that all exhaust fans are operating at the proper airflow.

(3) Increase the air-handling unit outdoor airflow until the building pressure relationship is positive 0.01 in. w.g. The building pressure relationship should be determined using a properly installed building pressure transmitter that measures the average differential pressure at the ground-level entrances to the building.

(4) Record the outdoor airflow, building pressure, and outdoor air temperature.

(5) If the outdoor airflow is excessive, the contractor should identify and seal envelope leaks.

(6) The testing and sealing process is then repeated until the amount of outdoor airflow is acceptable.

3.14 REVIEW RECORD DRAWINGS

The HFCxA should review the record drawings with O&M personnel. The HFCxA should identify known discrepancies between these documents and as-installed conditions. A list of these discrepancies is then forwarded to the owner, contractor, and design team for incorporation into the record documents.

Transition to
Operational Sustainability

4.1 FACILITATE DEVELOPMENT OF OPERATING AND MAINTENANCE DASHBOARDS

Many health care facilities have significantly reduced maintenance staffing levels and budgets in recent years. Staffing levels for skilled crafts and trades such as electricians, plumbers, HVAC technicians, and control instrument technicians are shockingly low. As a result, health care facility managers can no longer rely solely upon qualified staff to maintain complex equipment and systems. Rather, they must depend on technology to automatically detect inefficient operation and provide guidance for optimizing operation.

Dynamic operating and maintenance (O&M) dashboards created for the automatic temperature control system are well-suited for this purpose. Such dashboards have color-coded gauges (red—alarm, yellow—warning, and green—acceptable) to identify problems and sliders and knobs for adjusting set points and other control parameters.

4.1.1 Development of Dashboards

The HFCxA should facilitate development of O&M dashboards as specified in the owner's project requirements by working in conjunction with the design team, contractor, and controls contractor. (O&M dashboard requirements are included in the project design specifications, and the specifications for the sensors, meters, and control system integration they require are included in the contract documents and as part of the project scope.)

4.1.2 Systems Requiring Dashboards

The commissioning team should review the individual dashboards for compliance with the OPR and specified requirements. Dashboards should be included for the following:

(1) Building energy demands and costs. The energy dashboard should indicate actual building electricity, heating fuel, and water demands and costs as well as the current cost of building operation in dollars per hour.

(2) Air terminals. The air terminal dashboard should indicate the average terminal damper position, space temperature, discharge air temperature, heating valve position, and airflow as a percentage of maximum cooling airflow for each air-handling unit. This dashboard should also list all terminals with no airflow and open terminal dampers (indicating a failed airflow measuring device), terminals with closed heating water valves and high discharge air temperatures (indicating failed heating water valves), fully open terminal dampers, and fully open heating water valves.

(3) Air-handling units. Each air-handling unit should have its own dashboard. These dashboards should indicate supply airflow, supply fan speed, return fan speed, static pressure, supply air temperature, return air temperature, return air humidity, outside airflow in CFM, mixed air temperature, heating valve position, chilled water valve position, and humidifier valve position.

(4) Exhaust fan. The exhaust fan dashboard should indicate the operating status of each exhaust fan. It should also provide separate lists of exhaust fans that are not in operation when their associated air-handling unit is in operation and exhaust fans that are in operation when their associated air-handling unit is not in operation.

(5) Domestic hot water systems. Each domestic hot water system should have its own dashboard. These dashboards should indicate water heater flow, cold water flow, hot water supply temperature, hot water return temperature, cold water temperature, and the operating status of the recirculation pump.

(6) Heating water systems. Each heating water system should have its own dashboard. The dashboards should indicate heating water flow, heating water pump status, supply temperature, return temperature, temperature difference, heating water pump speed, differential pressure, and steam valve position.

(7) Chilled water system. The chilled water dashboard should indicate which water chillers are operating, the chilled water flow rate, supply

water temperature, return water temperature, temperature difference, total power requirement, average efficacy (kW/ton), pump operating status, pump speed, and differential pressure.

(8) Water chillers and cooling towers. The dashboards for this equipment should indicate equipment operating status, flow, entering and leaving water temperatures, and power consumption.

(9) Steam system. The steam dashboard should indicate which boilers are operating, the steam flow rate, make-up water flow rate, make-up water temperature, feedwater temperature, deaerator steam flow rate, fuel consumption, power consumption, and average fuel-to-steam efficiency.

(10) Boilers. The boiler dashboards should indicate equipment operating status, feedwater flow, feedwater temperature, steam flow, fuel flow, stack temperature, combustion efficiency, and power consumption.

(11) Fuel oil system. The fuel oil dashboard should indicate the fuel oil pump operating status and fuel oil storage level.

(12) Normal power system. The normal power system dashboard should indicate voltage, amps, apparent power, real power, power factor, and main breaker status.

(13) Essential power system. The essential power system dashboard should indicate which generators are operating and the automatic transfer switch positions.

4.2 FACILITATE MAINTENANCE STAFF TRAINING

4.2.1 Planning O&M Staff Training

Planning should be a topic in the early design stage of each project. Training requirements should be coordinated with the facility staff to ensure the planned level of training, schedule, and delivery will meet the needs of the staff. These criteria should be documented in the OPR and the training specifications should accommodate them. Further, the training specifications should require development of a detailed training program that defines how the training process will be executed.

The training program should be developed by the project construction team with support from manufacturers and vendors and should address the specific needs of the facility, such as coordination with multiple shifts. A detailed program should be documented and submitted to the design team, owner, and HFCxA for review and approval well before the training will be executed. The training program is then used as a guideline for scheduling and monitoring the training process.

The focus of the training process must be designed to meet the needs of the facility's O&M staff. Often, training is scheduled and executed at the convenience of vendors or contractors; the HFCxA should monitor scheduling and execution of the training process to make sure this does not occur. The HFCxA should also monitor the recordings made of the training process to ensure their quality is good enough for later training use. Training sessions (often 25 or more for a project) should be recorded by a professional service and stored in an "electronic library" format for easy access.

4.2.2 Testing Staff Knowledge

The HFCxA should also develop testing to assess the O&M staff's knowledge. Anonymous pre-testing is conducted prior to training to determine specific training needs. Anonymous post-testing is conducted afterward to verify the training's effectiveness and to identify additional training needs. Accrediting agencies require varying levels of documentation to show training comprehension on the part of the O&M staff. The HFCxA can develop test procedures that will provide this documentation as training occurs.

4.2.3 Training Program Components

(1) Instructor resumes

(2) A description of the general purpose of the equipment or system the training covers

(3) Use of the O&M manuals during the training process

(4) Material addressing these operational modes:

    (a) Start-up

    (b) Normal operation

    (c) Shutdown

    (d) Unoccupied operation

    (e) Seasonal changeover

    (f) Manual operation

    (g) Controls set-up and programming

    (h) Troubleshooting

    (i) Alarms

(5) Description of how the equipment/system interacts with other building systems and how it is included in operations dashboards

(6) Adjustments and optimizing methods for energy conservation

(7) Relevant health and safety issues

(8) Special maintenance and replacement sources

4.3 FACILITATE IMPLEMENTATION OF HVAC CONTROL SYSTEM TRENDS

The contract design scope should require creation of various trends to help the O&M staff monitor the operation of key equipment and systems in the facility. Often, the design documents require the HVAC control system to be capable of trending the systems but do not define the trends. In such cases, the HFCxA should assist the O&M staff in implementing key trends.

4.3.1 Purposes of Trending

Trends provide critical feedback on space conditions and energy usage. It is vitally important for O&M personnel to have this data to help them manage the facility and minimize energy costs. Trends can be implemented for various systems, but the focus should be on systems that have the most impact on energy usage and space conditions. Trends make it easier to diagnose control problems and identify system operations that are wasting energy or affecting space conditions and/or critical pressure relationships. Trends also identify how well control loops are tuned.

Review of trends after the building has been occupied is discussed in section 5.1 (Review Trend Data).

4.3.2 Trends to Consider for Development

Examples of trends that should be considered follow. Additional trends may be relevant depending on the specific needs of the facility.

(1) Terminal boxes and other zone control devices. Terminal boxes are either variable air volume (VAV) or constant volume (CAV) boxes. Trending terminal boxes can identify boxes that are performing incorrectly or wasting energy. Trends for similar criteria for other zone control devices (e.g., fan coil units, fan powered boxes, etc.) should also be defined. Trends for these types of equipment should monitor the following:

(a) Discharge air temperature

(b) Airflow

(c) Box damper position

(d) Thermostat set point

(e) Space temperature

(f) Reheat hot water valve position

(2) Heating hot water systems. Heating hot water systems should be controlled to minimize energy usage for pump horsepower and water temperature. The supply water temperature should be reset based on

load requirements and/or outside air temperature. The pumping system should be controlled based on demand (static pressure). Points that should be trended should include:

(a) Outside air temperature

(b) Supply and return water temperature

(c) Steam valve(s) position

(d) Differential pressure set point

(e) Actual static pressure at controlling sensor

(f) Pump speed and status

(g) System flow

(3) Air-handling units. Like terminal boxes, air-handling units (AHUs) are either VAV or CAV. They can serve one zone or multiple zones; be low, medium, or high pressure; and have chilled water coils, DX coils, or steam or hot water preheat or reheat coils (as well, some coils may have loop pumps). Air-handling units can have unit-mounted humidifiers and other associated equipment. Set points for supply air temperature and static pressure control should be reset based on load or outside air conditions. Points that should be trended include these:

(a) Supply air temperature and set point

(b) Airflows for supply, return, and outside air

(c) Static pressure set point and actual reading (may be multiple readings)

(d) Outside, return, and mixed air temperatures

(e) Control valve positions on the chilled water coils, preheat and reheat coils, and humidifier. The steam line to the humidifier should also have an automatic isolation valve that is monitored.

(f) Relative humidity reading in AHU supply air and at the space sensor

(g) Coil pump status (if applicable)

(h) Fan speed

(4) Chilled water system. The chilled water system (CHW) is usually the greatest energy load in the facility. It is also one that is most likely to operate inefficiently because of the criticality of the chilled water temperature and how it affects the supply air temperature in surgery and other mission critical areas. The two chilled water designs most

frequently used today are variable flow primary and primary/secondary systems. In addition, many designs include a water side economizer that utilizes various elements of the chilled water system to provide "free cooling." Each system contains numerous elements that must be monitored. Points that should be trended include these:

(a) Pump speeds for primary and secondary chilled water, condenser water pumps, plate and frame pumps

(b) Differential pressure set points and actual readings

(c) Water flows for primary and secondary chilled water, condenser water

(d) Chiller start/stops, chiller run time

(e) Outside air and water temperature set points and actual readings

(f) Isolation valves for chillers and cooling towers

(g) Cooling tower start/stops, fan speeds

4.4. PREPARE THE COMMISSIONING REPORT AND SYSTEMS MANUAL

4.4.1 Commissioning Report

The HFCxA completes the commissioning report and systems manual at the completion of the construction phase. The commissioning report summarizes and documents the methodology and results of the commissioning process and includes documentation of all commissioning activities. The report generally includes:

(1) An executive summary (This should summarize the process and the results of the commissioning process.)

(2) A history of the action items and deficiencies noted and how they were resolved

(3) System performance tests and evaluations

(4) A summary of the design review and submittal processes

(5) A summary of the O&M documentation and training processes

(6) Commissioning documentation from throughout the process, including

(a) Meeting minutes

(b) Completed documents such as start-up documents, completed prefunctional checklists, functional performance test results, training data, and so on.

4.4.2 Systems Manual

The HFCxA also compiles the systems manual, which focuses on operating systems. One of the most important uses for this document is as a condensed system-level troubleshooting guide for O&M personnel. At minimum, the systems manual should include the following:

(1) Final version of the OPR and BOD

(2) System single-line drawings

(3) As-built sequences of operation

(4) Control shop drawings

(5) Original control set points

(6) Operating instructions for integrated systems

(7) Recommended retesting schedule and blank test forms

(8) Sensor and actuator recalibration schedules

4.5 FACILITATE DEVELOPMENT OF THE MAINTENANCE BUDGET

The HFCxA should ensure that the health care administrative staff and facility manager have an accurate and thorough understanding of the resources needed to maintain and operate the health care facility in a cost-effective manner (e.g., staffing, materials, service contracts, etc.). The recommended staffing level and maintenance budget for the facility should be determined using the ASHE benchmarking tool, which bases its recommendations on facility age, floor areas, labor rates, Energy Star rating, weather, and the specific maintenance services provided by in-house personnel and outsourced service contracts. Figure 2-3 shows a sample output prepared using the tool.

ASHE created its benchmarking tool from data collected directly from hospitals. Unlike other benchmarking methods, which are somewhat arbitrary in nature, the ASHE tool considers site-specific information. Figure 2-4 shows staffing levels and maintenance and operating costs for four different sizes and types of

Item	Recommended Amount ($/year)
Staffing	3,256,696
Education	65,134
Tools	32,567
Materials	1,115,870
Service contracts	767,810
Utilities	11,797,452
Total	17,035,529
Unit cost ($/sq. ft.)	4.72

Figure 2-3: Sample ASHE Maintenance Benchmarking Tool Output

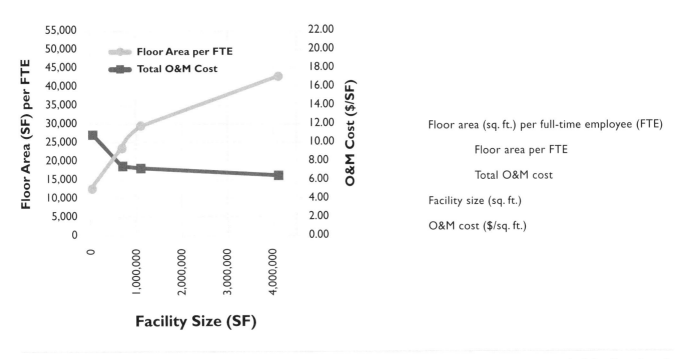

Floor area (sq. ft.) per full-time employee (FTE)

Floor area per FTE

Total O&M cost

Facility size (sq. ft.)

O&M cost ($/sq. ft.)

Figure 2-4: Health Care Facility Recommended Staffing Levels

hospitals; this data is the average of input from facilities that participated in development of the ASHE benchmarking tool.

The costs and staffing levels indicated in Figure 2-4 include grounds, but do not include data management, compliance, housekeeping, biomedical equipment maintenance, or security. The staffing levels vary from 12,000 square feet per FTE for a small 100,000-square-foot facility up to 42,000 square feet per FTE for a massive 4 million-square-foot facility. The maintenance and operating costs (including energy costs) vary inversely from $11 per square foot for the smaller facility down to $7 per square foot for the larger facility. The vast difference between the smaller and larger facilities suggests that other simplified benchmarking approaches may not yield useful or actionable results.

4.6 FACILITATE FIRE AND SMOKE DAMPER INSPECTIONS AND TESTING

4.6.1 Code Requirements

National codes require health care facilities to inspect and test their fire and smoke dampers within 12 months of installation and every six years thereafter. To reduce costs and minimize disruption, the HFCxA should work with the contractor to complete the initial damper inspection and testing at the completion of the construction phase, immediately before the building is occupied.

Provide a written report listing each damper number, damper location, date of inspection, damper inspection results, and associated corrective work, if required. The HFCxA should forward a final approved copy of this report to the facility manager.

4.6.2 Scope for Damper Inspection and Testing

Work items should include the following:

(1) Verify that the record drawings accurately indicate the location of all fire and smoke dampers and that the dampers are properly labeled.

(2) Locate all fire and smoke dampers. Verify that the dampers are properly tagged.

(3) Remove and reset fusible links on fire dampers to verify each damper fully closes. Replace fusible links as required.

(4) Lubricate all moving parts on each damper.

(5) Clear each damper of any obstruction impeding the dampers' normal operation.

(6) Manually activate each smoke damper and combination fire-and smoke-damper actuator to verify proper operation.

4.7 FACILITATE COMPLETION OF THE STATEMENT OF CONDITIONS (SOC)

In addition to the utility management plan (UMP), the Joint Commission accreditation process requires development of the Statement of Conditions (SOC). Where applicable, the HFCxA should work with the owner and the design team to facilitate completion of the SOC for the building.

4.8 FACILITATE DEVELOPMENT AND IMPLEMENTATION OF THE BUILDING MAINTENANCE PROGRAM (BMP)

4.8.1 Timing and Software Requirement

After the design is completed and well in advance of project completion and occupancy, the HFCxA should work with the facility manager, design team, and contractor to develop and implement a building maintenance program (BMP) for new facilities or update the existing BMP for renovations and additions. The BMP should utilize a computerized maintenance management system (CMMS) software program.

4.8.2 HFCxA Scope

The scope of the HFCxA's involvement in the development and implementation of the maintenance management program should include the following items of work:

(1) Ensure that all equipment is numbered and labeled in a manner consistent with facility standards. For renovation and addition projects, the equipment numbers should begin with the next available number (not start over again at 1).

(2) Ensure that room numbers indicated on the construction drawings are consistent with facility standards and actual room numbers. The actual room numbers are frequently different from the room numbers indicated on the construction drawings; this inconsistency wreaks havoc on the O&M staff and poses a significant barrier to achieving an effective transition from construction completion to sustainable operation.

(3) Ensure the owner receives an electronic archive of all information required to operate and maintain the facility. If possible, the design team and contractor should insert the electronic archive into a three-dimensional electronic model of the building (a building information model, sometimes called a BIM). The archive should include the following:

   (a) Design calculations

   (b) Record drawings

   (c) Project manual

   (d) Submittals

   (e) Shop drawings

   (f) Coordination drawing

   (g) Factory test reports

   (g) Pre-functional checklists

   (h) Equipment start-up reports

   (i) TAB reports

   (j) Functional performance test results

   (k) Other test results

   (l) Installation requirements

   (m) Operations and maintenance manuals

      (n) Spare parts inventory

      (o) Recommended schedule and frequency for maintenance procedures

      (p) Parts lists

      (q) Warranties

      (r) Service contracts

      (s) Service provider contact information

(4) Ensure each item of equipment and its associated maintenance and operating information is identified in the CMMS.

(5) Ensure the CMMS automatically generates work orders for recommended maintenance procedures at the recommended frequency.

(6) Ensure a complete service history for each item of equipment (scheduled maintenance, unscheduled maintenance, etc.) is maintained in the CMMS.

(7) Ensure the CMMS provides for regular (annual or more frequent) calibration of temperature, pressure, and other sensors critical to efficient system performance.

Postoccupancy and Warranty Phase

5.1 REVIEW TREND DATA

In section 4.3 (Implement HVAC Control System Trends), the implementation of automatic temperature control trends was discussed. When the facility is occupied and the systems are subjected to actual load conditions, trends provide the facility manager with critical data that allow him or her to optimize system operations for both building comfort and energy management. Vital real-time feedback can be obtained by integrating trend data into the O&M dashboards. The HFCxA can assist the staff in interpreting the trend data and in optimizing performance.

5.1.1 Terminal Boxes

Trending the operation of terminal boxes will identify problems such as these:

(1) Simultaneous heating and cooling—The performance of the air side can be compared to the reheat valve control to ensure the airflow varies as required prior to actually calling for reheat.

(2) Malfunctioning box dampers and reheat hot water control valves—Boxes may be programmed incorrectly, allowing the control signal to call for the valve or damper to close when, in fact, the devices are opening. This is readily apparent from the readings in the trend.

(3) Blockages in the heating water piping system—Blockages can be readily diagnosed from discharge air temperature readings when the box is calling for heat. Blockages can be caused by trash in the lines or an isolation valve that is closed. Also the piping may be partially blocked as would be noted by an inadequate heat gain across the heating coil.

(4) Capability of the boxes to satisfy space temperature—The space temperature set point should be maintained at all times by the terminal box. Trending will identify a system's ability to maintain set point.

(5) Excessive energy use from "over-airing" the space—Monitoring airflows against the sequence of operation will determine whether the box resets to the specified airflows as conditions change in the space.

5.1.2 Heating Hot Water System (HWS)

Trending the heating hot water system will identify problems such as these:

(1) Outside air and supply water temperature—The heating water temperature should be reset based on the outside air temperature. Trending will determine whether the heating water supply temperature set point is being properly controlled.

(2) Supply and return water temperatures—The system is designed for a temperature drop across the system. Monitoring the supply and return water temperature differential and the system water flow will indicate the system's ability to meet the demand of the load.

(3) Steam valve(s) position—The position of the steam valve will indicate how well the control loop is tuned and the steam system's ability to serve the load. The valve should modulate to maintain set point and not be 100 percent open at all times. If more than one steam valves serves a system, the valves should be different sizes so the smaller valve operates during minimal load conditions to provide better control of the HWS temperature.

(4) Differential pressure, set point and actual reading, and pump speed—Pump speed should vary as the load varies. The set point should be sufficient to meet the load demands but not so high that the pump operates at excessive speeds. Trending will also indicate how well the control loop is tuned.

(5) Pump status—Pumps are programmed to operate in series or in parallel, depending on the design. Trends will indicate when pumps are being operated excessively.

5.1.3 Air-Handling Units (AHUs)

Trending the AHUs will identify problems such as these:

(1) Static pressure—Does the system maintain the static pressure set point? Does the fan speed modulate or are the VFDs at 100 percent most of the time? Are the control loops tuned?

(2) Simultaneous heating and cooling—Does simultaneous heating and cooling occur between the cooling coils and heating coils?

(3) Humidifier—Does the humidifier maintain set point? Does the relative humidity (RH) in the supply duct remain safely below the saturation point? Is the humidifier turned off when not needed?

(4) Fan tracking—In variable volume systems, the relationship between supply, return, and outside airflows is critical to maintaining the appropriate building pressure relationship. The fans must track as the load varies. Both negatively pressurized facilities and overly positive facilities will experience significant performance issues.

(5) Coil pumps—These pumps should only operate when designated to do so. They reduce the risk of coil freezing and damage, but—if operating incorrectly—can be a source of wasted energy.

(6) Control valves—The valve positions will indicate how well the load is matched to the coils. Do the valve positions modulate with the load? Are the control loops tuned?

5.1.4 Chilled Water System (CHW)

Chillers should be controlled in conjunction with the condenser water system and pumping system to meet load requirements while minimizing energy usage. Generally, chillers operate more efficiently when fully loaded; thus, it is critical to load them and maintain the load side water temperature differential. Chiller manufacturers offer integration panels that share chiller performance information with the building automation system. This data-sharing allows the facility manger to optimize system performance and monitor critical performance criteria in the chillers. Trending the chilled water system will identify problems such as these:

(1) Chiller loading—Is the overall system being operated to maintain maximum load on the chillers? If multiple partially loaded chillers are being operated, the controls and load side conditions should be investigated.

(2) Chiller stops and starts—Chillers should not have excessive starts. Proper loading of chillers and a well-defined control sequence for adding and dropping chillers based on the connected load will minimize starts. If trending indicates multiple starts, system lead/lag controls should be investigated.

(3) Chiller runtime—Assuming all the chillers in a plant are equally efficient, chiller runtime should be shared to ensure the chillers are operated equally. Often, chillers have differing efficiencies or different

sizes. These parameters will dictate the sequence for starting and stopping chillers as the load varies. Chillers of equal efficiencies and sizes should have equal runtime.

(4) Primary CHW flow vs. secondary CHW flow—In primary/secondary systems, the primary flow should be greater than the secondary flow to prohibit mixing return with supply water. Trending will indicate if the system ever experiences a load condition where mixing occurs.

(5) Primary CHW temperature vs. secondary CHW temperature—In primary/secondary systems, the design primary loop temperature differential should be less than or equal to the secondary loop temperature differential. If the differential is less in the secondary system, it will not allow the chillers to load properly. Trending will indicate if the system ever experiences a load condition where the primary loop temperature differential is greater than that in the secondary.

(6) Differential pressure, set point and actual reading, and pump speed—Pump speed should vary as the load varies. The set point should be adequate to meet the load demands, but not so high as to operate the pump at excessive speeds. Trending will indicate how well the control loop is tuned.

5.1.5 Other Equipment

Trending the cooling tower fan speed and condenser water supply and return temperatures will identify optimal operation. Water should be distributed over the full capacity of a multiple cell tower before operating tower fans. Modulating tower controls to match the optimal condenser water supply temperature will optimize chiller efficiency.

5.2 MEASURE AND VERIFY ACTUAL ENERGY PERFORMANCE

After the project is complete, the HFCxA should work with the facility manager to establish a Portfolio Manager account on the EPA Energy Star website and enter the required building information, which includes floor areas, parking decks, data centers, pools, and bed count.

The facility manager should enter actual electricity, heating fuel, and water consumption and costs into the Portfolio Manager account. These figures should be compared each month to the consumption and costs predicted by the previously developed energy model (see section 2.2 (Set Project Energy Efficiency Goals). If the actual consumption and costs exceed the predicted levels, the HFCxA should work with the facility manager, design team, and contractor to identify the cause of the disparity and implement corrective action.

The facility will receive a baseline Energy Star rating when the Portfolio Manager account includes 12 months of data. If the actual Energy Star rating is less than the target Energy Star rating, the HFCxA should again work with the facility manager, design team, and contractor to identify the cause of the disparity and implement corrective action.

To ensure that health care facility administrative and maintenance staff remain vigilant regarding energy efficiency, the HFCxA should assist the facility manager with development of an energy efficiency scorecard. The facility manager should publish the scorecard each month. See Figure 2-5 for a sample energy efficiency scorecard.

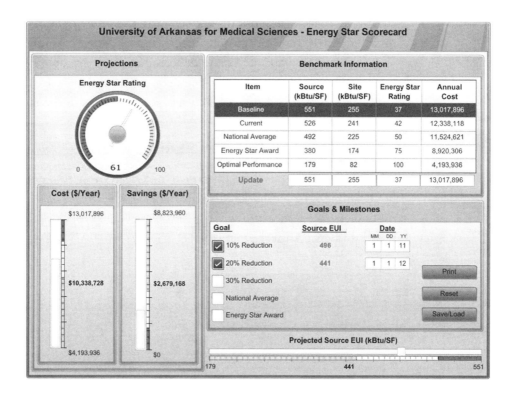

Figure 2-5: Sample Energy Efficiency Scorecard

5.3 CONDUCT POSTOCCUPANCY PERFORMANCE TESTS

The completion of a project rarely coincides with peak load conditions related to the local climate, but it is necessary to functionally test systems under peak loads within the warranty period. Generally, there are two seasonal peak load times (peak winter and summer). The HFCxA must coordinate required seasonal or deferred testing and follow up noted deficiencies until corrections are made. A report documenting this testing process should be included in the commissioning record.

The testing is focused on documenting functionality related to the conditions dictated by the appropriate season. For example, humidifiers and water and air side economizers can only be adequately tested during the winter season. Peak load capacities on chilled water systems can only be adequately tested during summer peak periods. Functional testing of safeties, alarms, and emergency power systems not impacted by the seasons should be conducted prior to occupancy.

5.4 PARTICIPATE IN THE END-OF-WARRANTY REVIEW

The HFCxA participates with the owner, contractor, and design team in a comprehensive review of the project near the end of the warranty phase (8 to 10 months after substantial completion). The review identifies outstanding construction deficiencies and deficiencies discovered by the operations and maintenance staff. The HFCxA assists other members of the project team with correction of deficiencies and reports outcomes to the facility manager.

5.5 BENCHMARK ENERGY PERFORMANCE

After the building has been in service for a year, the actual energy efficiency of the building is benchmarked by the owner or the HFCxA. The benchmarking process is based on actual energy and water consumption and costs as compared to the EPA target.

Retrocommissioning

6.1 THE RETROCOMMISSIONING PROCESS

6.1.1 Who Leads the Effort

Retrocommissioning efforts should be led by a HFCxA. The HFCxA should work in conjunction with O&M personnel to optimize building performance.

6.1.2 Items of Work for Retrocommissioning Energy-Consuming Systems

The retrocommissioning process for energy-consuming systems in health care facilities should include these items of work:

(1) Establish an Energy Star Portfolio Manager account for the health care facility.

(2) Obtain 24 months of natural gas, water, and electricity bills and enter them into the Portfolio Manager account.

(3) Enter other required facility data into the Portfolio Manager account. Obtain a baseline Energy Star rating for the facility.

(4) Establish a target Energy Star rating for the facility.

(5) Identify the potential energy cost savings associated with increasing the Energy Star rating from the baseline level to the target level.

(6) Obtain and review construction drawings and specifications for the original construction and any renovations to the facility.

(7) Obtain and review major equipment submittal data for the original construction and renovations.

(8) Obtain and review TAB reports for the original construction and renovations.

(9) Obtain and review control diagrams for the original construction and renovations.

(10) Conduct a detailed survey of the facility with a focus on the mechanical rooms, electrical rooms, and energy-consuming equipment and systems (water chillers, boilers, water heaters, air-handling units, exhaust fans, and pumps).

(11) Conduct a detailed review of automatic temperature control systems, including water chillers, boilers, air terminals, air-handling units, exhaust fans, domestic water heating equipment, and fan coil units. Identify existing sequences of operation and set points.

(12) Obtain and evaluate utility rate structures for natural gas, electricity, and water. Identify and evaluate potential supply-side measures to reduce energy costs.

(13) Identify and evaluate demand-side energy cost reduction opportunities. Develop estimates of implementation cost, annual savings, and simple payback for each demand-side energy cost reduction opportunity.

(14) Discuss supply-side and demand-side energy cost reduction opportunities with the facility manager. Develop a long-range plan to implement changes proposed to reduce energy expenditures and costs.

(15) Develop a scorecard to track and record actual energy cost savings (progress toward reaching the energy cost reduction target).

(16) Conduct detailed testing of water chillers and chilled water pumps. Measure and record pressures, temperatures, flows, and power consumption.

(17) Conduct detailed testing of boilers and heating water pumps. Measure and record pressures, temperatures, flows, and power consumption.

(18) Conduct detailed testing of each large air-handling unit. Measure and record outside airflow, return airflow, and supply airflow. Measure and record static pressure drops in each section. Measure and record dry bulb and wet bulb temperatures in each section. Measure and record fan speeds, fan motor currents, and fan motor electrical demand.

(19) Conduct detailed testing of each large exhaust fan. Measure and record airflow, fan static pressure, fan speed, fan motor current, and fan motor electrical demand.

(20) Compare actual equipment performance to manufacturer's rated performance data. Identify and document discrepancies.

(21) Establish and review trends for key equipment operating parameters.

(22) Develop a detailed room ventilation schedule for the facility. The schedule should identify floor area, ceiling height, room volume, outdoor air change requirement, total air change requirement, pressure relationships, existing airflow set points, and proposed airflow set points.

(23) Develop weekly occupied/unoccupied or on/off schedules for air-handling units and other equipment.

(24) Develop revised air-handling unit sequences of operation and set points for optimum energy efficiency (supply air temperature control, humidity control, economizer cycles, damper sequencing, supply air temperature setpoint reset, and supply air static pressure set point reset).

(25) Establish revised air-handling unit outside airflow set points.

(26) Establish revised exhaust fan airflow requirements.

(27) Establish revised chilled water and heating water system sequences of operation for optimum energy efficiency (temperature set point reset, differential pressure set point reset, pump speed control and sequencing, etc.).

(28) Establish weekly occupied/unoccupied or on/off schedules for air terminals and fan coil units. Establish unoccupied heating and cooling set points.

(29) Establish revised air terminal sequences of operation for optimum energy efficiency.

(30) Establish revised fan coil unit sequences of operation for optimum energy efficiency.

(31) Establish revised air terminal airflow set points (eight settings).

(32) Establish minimum and maximum limits for thermostat set points.

(33) Establish revised deadband settings for space heating and cooling set points.

(34) Document the work in a written report.

6.1.3 Striving for Continuous Commissioning®

The use of an electronic commissioning tool that interfaces with the automatic temperature control system can significantly expedite the retrocommissioning effort. The tool uses a standard communication protocol to query a massive database and quickly identify previously undetected problem areas. After the retrocommissioning effort is completed, O&M staff can use the tool to continuously identify problems and dispatch maintenance personnel. The retro-commissioning effort should lead toward the implementation of a continuous commissioning effort that is appropriate for the specific facility.

6.2 RETROCOMMISSIONING CASE STUDIES

Retrocommissioning health care facilities can significantly reduce annual energy costs. An acute care hospital located in Fort Scott, Kansas, opened in 2003 and operated in an "as-constructed" state until 2005, when the health care organization initiated retrocommissioning work. The result of the facility's retrocommissioning effort is illustrated in Figure 2-6.

Item	Before	After	Savings (%)	Remarks
Electricity consumption (kWh)	7,808,800	5,249,800	32.8	
Average peak demand (kW)	1,230	929	24.5	
Electricity consumption (kWh/sq. ft./year)	44.0	29.6	32.8	Mercy average is 32 kWh/sq. ft./year.
Average peak demand (watts/sq. ft.)	6.93	5.23	24.5	
Natural gas consumption (MMBtu)	43,114	23,523	45.4	
Natural gas consumption (therms/sq. ft./year)	2.43	1.33	45.4	Mercy average is 1.23 therms/sq. ft./year.
Total energy consumption (MMBtu)	70,137	41,457	40.90	
Energy utilization index (kBtu/sq. ft.)	393	233	40.6	Mercy average is 232 kBtu/sq. ft./year.
Total energy cost ($/year)	916,182	540,058	41.1	
Energy cost index ($/sq. ft./year)	5.16	3.04	41.1	Mercy average is $2.85/sq. ft.

Figure 2-6: Sample Retrocommissioning Results from Fort Scott

As indicated in the figure, the hospital reduced its annual energy costs by more than 40 percent without compromising thermal comfort, system reliability, or infection control. The retrocommissioning effort identified and corrected the HVAC system problems listed on the next page:

- The minimum cooling and minimum heating air terminal airflow set points had been set at the same levels as the maximum cooling and maximum heating airflow set points.

- The air terminals, exhaust fans, and air-handling units did not have defined occupied/unoccupied schedules.

- The air-handling unit sequences of operation provided for simultaneous humidification and air-side economizer cycle operation.

- The air-handling unit sequences of operation provided for simultaneous operation of the preheat coils and the chilled water coils (set points overlapped).

- The air-handling unit supply air temperature and supply air static pressure control programs did not include any type of set point reset.

- One of the cooling tower fan motors was undersized, causing condenser water supply temperatures during warm weather to exceed 90 deg. F.

- Manual balancing valves located in the discharge piping of the chilled water, condenser water, and heating water pumps had been partially closed to balance flow rates to design levels (instead of slowing down the pump speeds using variable frequency drives).

The primary driving force behind the energy savings was the adjustment of the air terminal set points. Figure 2-7 illustrates the "as-constructed" air terminal sequence of operation in the graph on the left and the air terminal sequence of operation after the retrocommissioning effort in the graph on the right. A comparison of the two graphs clearly indicates the substantial reduction in airflow and simultaneous heating and cooling achieved by the retrocommissioning work.

A cardiovascular hospital located in Oklahoma City opened in 2004 and operated in an "as-constructed" state until 2006, when the health care organization initiated a retrocommissioning effort.

As indicated in Figure 2-8, which illustrates the results of the Oklahoma City retrocommissioning effort, the hospital reduced its annual energy cost by nearly 30 percent. The issues discovered and corrected at this facility were very similar to those at the Fort Scott facility. The retrocommissioning effort at Oklahoma City also reduced the facility's peak chilled water, steam, heating water, and electricity loads to the extent that the existing systems, without modification, were able to accommodate a 50 percent increase in floor area without sacrificing reliability or redundancy.

The simple payback in both of these retrocommissioning case studies was considerably less than one year, demonstrating the cost-effectiveness of retrocommissioning existing facilities.

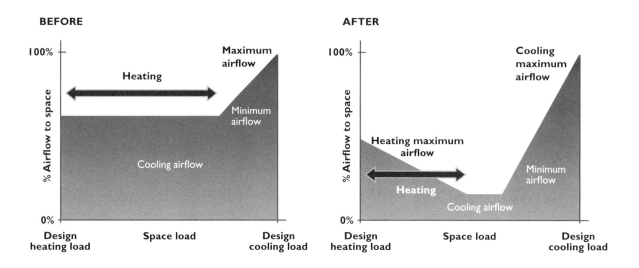

Figure 2-7: Air Terminal Operation Before and After Retrocommissioning

Item	Before	After	Savings (%)	Remarks
Electricity consumption (kWh)	10,175,200	8,884,600	12.7	
Average peak demand (kW)	1,499	1,403	6.4	
Electricity consumption (kWh/sq. ft./year)	49.9	43.6	12.7	Mercy average is 32 kWh/sq. ft./year.
Electricity load factor (%)	77	72	6.7	
Average peak demand (watts/sq. ft.)	7.3	6.9	6.4	
Natural gas consumption (MMBtu)	35,507	28,283	20.3	
Natural gas consumption (therms/sq. ft./year)	1.7	1.4	20.3	Mercy average is 1.23 therms/sq. ft./year.
Total energy consumption (MMBtu)	70,235	58,606	16.6	
Energy utilization index (kBtu/sq. ft.)	396	330	16.6	Mercy average is 232 kBtu/sq. ft./year.
Total energy cost ($/year)	1,121,614	801,141	28.6	
Energy cost index ($/sq. ft./year)	5.50	3.93	28.6	Mercy average is $2.85/sq. ft.

Figure 2-8: Sample Retrocommissioning Results from Oklahoma City

APPENDICES

Sample Commissioning RFP

SOLICITATION FOR COMMISSIONING SERVICES

(Owner)
(Project Name)
(Location)

(Date)

Background

(**Owner**) is seeking the services of a qualified Health Facility Commissioning Authority (HFCxA) for a new health care construction project. The project is a (**Project description, including current status and schedule**).

The project is presently in the design phase. Construction is anticipated to begin in (**Month-year**) and to be completed in (**Month-year**).

The design of the project is by (**Architect and/or Engineer**). (**Construction Manager Firm Name**) is the Construction Manager. The HFCxA will report to the Owner. The Owner's Representative is:

(*Owner's Rep Name*)
(*Title-if applicable*)
(*Company*)
(*Address*)
(*City, ST ZIP*)

Scope of work

The primary role of the HFCxA is to ensure that the Owner's Project Requirements (OPR) are developed during the planning phase and are achieved through the design, construction, and operation of the facility.

The following is a summary of the commissioning process the Owner intends to have implemented on this project. This process is as defined in the ASHE *Health Facility Commissioning Guidelines*. For this proposal, the following process will be followed.

I. COMMISSIONING PROCESS

A. Commissioning Process during Design

   1) Meetings

      a) Predesign conference—The HFCxA will organize and attend a predesign conference at the beginning of the Design Phase. The HFCxA will prepare an agenda for the meeting that addresses the project goals, scope, team member responsibilities, delivery process, project budget, schedule, and performance expectations.

      b) Design review meetings—The HFCxA will be required to attend the design review meetings at the end of each design phase (SD, DD, CD). The meetings will be held at the (Architect's **complete as appropriate**) office in (*City, State*).

   2) Owner's project requirements (OPR)—The HFCxA will facilitate development of the OPR. The Owner, design team, and HFCxA will work collaboratively to develop the OPR.

      a) The HFCxA will work with the Owner, design team, and contractor or third-party project manager hired by the Owner to establish an aggressive yet attainable and fiscally responsible energy efficiency goal.

      b) The HFCxA will chair an OPR charrette and prepare an agenda for the charrette that covers all elements of the OPR as defined in the ASHE *Health Facility Commissioning Guidelines*.

      c) The HFCxA will prepare a draft of the OPR from the minutes of the OPR charrette for for final review and comment by the participants. The HFCxA will prepare a final OPR based on the draft review comments. The HFCxA will modify the OPR as the project progresses through the design and construction phases.

   3) Commissioning specifications

      a) The HFCxA will develop full commissioning specifications based on the OPR.

b) The HFCxA will coordinate with the design team to integrate the commissioning specifications into the project specifications prepared by the project architect and engineers.

c) The commissioning specifications will include the elements defined in the ASHE *Health Facility Commissioning Guidelines*, including a detailed description of the responsibilities of all the parties, details of the commissioning process, reporting and documentation requirements (including formats), deficiency resolution, pre-functional checklist requirements, functional testing requirements, test and balancing requirements, training, O&M manuals, record document requirements, and retesting responsibilities.

4) Design documents—The HFCxA will review the design documents with a focus on commissionability, design completeness, cost-effectiveness, coordination of trades, and energy efficiency. HFCxA will include the hospital O&M staff in this review. For each review, the HFCxA will prepare a written list of comments for the Owner and design team. The HFCxA will conduct the following reviews:

a) Basis of design (BOD)—Review the BOD to verify compliance with the OPR. The design engineer is to provide the BOD documentation for use during this review.

b) Plan reviews—Perform reviews at 100% completion of schematic design documents (SDs), design development documents (DDs), and construction documents (CDs).

c) HVAC control system sequences of operation—Review these sequences carefully to make certain they contain adequate detail and incorporate energy-efficient processes (e.g., static pressure set point reset, supply air temperature set point reset, occupancy sensors, unoccupied/occupied air changes rates, weekly scheduling with optimal start/stop, etc.).

5) Utility management plan (UMP)—The HFCxA will facilitate the development of the UMP. The HFCxA will work with the facility manager, design team, and contractor to facilitate development of the plan prior to completion of the final design. The UMP will include all the components as outlined in the ASHE *Health Facility Commissioning Guidelines*.

6) Commissioning plan—The HFCxA will develop a commissioning plan that encompasses the design, construction, and occupancy and operations phases. In the design phase, the HFCxA will develop the initial commissioning plan, including the following:

a) A project-specific description of equipment to be commissioned

b) A description of the roles of the HFCx team, including the responsibilities of the Owner, A/E, contractors, and HFCxA

c) Sample prototypical pre-functional checklists (PFCs) for each piece of equipment in the commissioning scope

d) Sample prototypical functional performance tests (FPTs) that define acceptable results of the tests to be performed

B. Commissioning Process During Construction and Acceptance Phases

1) Meetings

a) Kick-off meeting—The HFCxA will plan and conduct a pre-construction commissioning meeting within 60 days of contract award.

b) Commissioning meetings—The HFCxA will coordinate and direct the commissioning activities in conjunction with the contractor and/or construction manager in a logical, sequential, and efficient manner using consistent protocols, clear and regular communications and consultations with all necessary parties, frequently updated timelines and schedules, and technical expertise. Meetings will be held as necessary to coordinate the commissioning process. At minimum, the HFCxA will conduct "milestone meetings" at the beginning of each phase of commissioning, including the following:

   i. Shop drawing submission
   ii. Equipment installation
   iii. Creation of pre-functional checklists
   iv. Equipment start-up
   v. Functional performance testing
   vi. Submission of operating and maintenance manuals
   vii. Owner training
   viii. Seasonal testing
   ix. One-year warranty testing

c) Project meetings—The HFCxA will review the minutes of the regular project meetings and attend selected project meetings as needed to resolve issues and concerns and coordinate the commissioning process.

2) Construction phase commissioning plan—The HFCxA will revise the commissioning plan developed during design, including scope and schedule, as necessary.

a) The HFCxA will prepare project-specific pre-functional checklists (PFCs) for each piece of equipment in the commissioning scope and include these in the commissioning plan. Generic PFCs or equipment start-up checklists are not acceptable.

b) Prepare project-specific functional performance test (FPT) procedures that define acceptable results of the tests to be performed and include these in the commissioning plan. Generic FPTs are not acceptable.

3) Reviews

a) Shop drawings—The HFCxA will review contractor submittals applicable to systems being commissioned to ensure compliance with the commissioning plan, commissioning specifications, and OPR. The HFCxA also reviews these documents with facility O&M personnel. The HFCxA will forward comments and concerns in writing to the design team and the Owner. Reviews must be concurrent with A/E reviews, must be conducted in a timely manner, and must not affect the construction schedule of the contractor.

b) O&M manuals—The HFCxA shall review the manuals to ensure proper content and format.

c) Start-up plan—The HFCxA will review the start-up plan to ensure operational parameters outlined in the OPR will be met. The review will include start-up training procedures for maintenance personnel who will be operating the equipment after occupancy.

d) HVAC control system programming—The HFCxA will review the programs before implementation and again after implementation to ensure proper performance of the HVAC system.

e) Training program—The HFCxA will review training procedures for all equipment included in the commissioning plan to ensure an appropriate transition to operational sustainability by maintenance personnel. These training procedures should be specific to the unique parameters the O&M staff will need to manage to ensure the equipment performs at the desired efficiencies outlined in the OPR. These training procedures are in addition to standard training in systems operation normally associated with turnover/takeover activities at the end of a project.

f) TAB report—The HFCxA will review the testing, adjusting, and balancing (TAB) report prepared by the contractor and prepare a written response. The HFCxA will also spot-check a representative sample of airflow and water flow readings as documented in the TAB report. The duration of the sampling will be two eight-hour days.

g) Record drawings—The HFCxA will review the record drawings with O&M personnel and identify known discrepancies between these documents and as-installed conditions. The HFCxA will forward a list of these discrepancies to the Owner, contractor, and design team for incorporation into the record documents.

4) Scheduling—The HFCxA will coordinate the commissioning tasks with the general contractor (GC) and construction manager (CM) to ensure that commissioning activities are included in their master schedule. The HFCxA will develop a testing plan for all equipment, systems, and integrated systems.

5) O&M staff construction site tours—The HFCxA will lead facility O&M personnel on regular tours of the construction site, discussing the equipment, systems, OPR, BOD, scheduled maintenance requirements, sequences of operation, and so on. The HFCxA maintains a list of O&M staff comments and concerns and works with the contractor and design team to respond to these.

6) Pre-functional inspections and checklists—The HFCxA will execute the PFCs in phases (e.g., equipment installation, piping rough-in, electrical rough-in, controls rough-in, feeder and load side termination for electrical systems, etc.) as the work progresses. The purpose of this process is to document that installation occurs per the contract documents as the work is installed rather than waiting until all installation is complete. Resolution of deficiencies is documented on subsequent site visits. All elements of equipment and system installation and all PFCs must be complete prior to functional testing.

7) Equipment and systems start-up—The HFCxA reviews equipment start-up procedures, witnesses the start-up of critical systems, and reviews the completed start-up documentation.

8) Functional performance tests—The HFCxA will direct execution of the functional performance tests by the responsible subcontractors. The FPTs are conducted at design full load, part load, and emergency conditions. The tests proceed from tests of simple system to tests of complex system to tests of integrated systems. The HFCxA invites O&M personnel to attend and witness testing. The HFCxA documents test results and recommends systems for acceptance.

   a) Facilitate pressure testing—Per ASHE *Health Facility Commissioning Guidelines* requirements, pressure testing will be conducted on isolation rooms and associated anterooms, operating rooms, procedure rooms, airborne infection isolation (AII) rooms, and protective environment (PE) rooms.

   b) Fire and smoke damper testing—The HFCxA will verify that all dampers have been tested per the ASHE *Health Facility Commissioning Guidelines* and provide a report (as defined in those guidelines) that lists each damper number, damper location, date of inspection, and damper inspection results.

    c) The HFCxA will functionally test O&M dashboards and document the accuracy of the data they report.

    d) The HFCxA will document that specified trends are implemented and operational as required by the commissioning specifications.

9) Site visits—The HFCxA will perform site visits, as necessary, to observe component and system installations.

    a) Maintain a master issues log and separate testing record. The log will include a definition of each issue, the date it was identified, a proposed corrective plan, the responsible party, the date of anticipated resolution, and its current status.

    b) Provide the Owner with written progress reports and test results with recommended actions.

10) Training

    a) The HFCxA will monitor scheduling and execution of the training process to ensure it is conducted as specified and as planned in the training program. The HFCxA will also monitor recordings made of the training process to ensure their quality is acceptable according to specifications.

    b) The HFCxA will develop testing to assess the O&M staff's knowledge.

11) Final commissioning report and systems manual. The HFCxA will complete the commissioning report and a systems manual for turnover/takeover at the completion of the construction phase. These documents will conform to the requirements of the ASHE *Health Facility Commissioning Guidelines*.

C. Commissioning During the Occupancy and Operation Phases

1) Maintenance budget—The HFCxA will facilitate development of the facility's maintenance budget. The recommended staffing level and maintenance budget for the facility should be determined using benchmarking tools such as those defined in the ASHE *Health Facility Commissioning Guidelines*.

2) Maintenance program—The HFCxA will facilitate development of the facility's maintenance program. The scope of the HFCxA's involvement in the development and implementation of the maintenance management program will be as recommended in the ASHE *Health Facility Commissioning Guidelines*.

3) Testing—Coordinate required seasonal or deferred testing and deficiency corrections and provide final testing documentation for the commissioning record and O&M manuals.

4) Postoccupancy visits—The HFCxA will return to the site 10 months into the 12-month warranty period and review with facility staff the current building operation and the condition of outstanding issues related to the original and seasonal commissioning. Also interview facility staff and identify problems or concerns they have with operating the building as originally intended.

5) Documents to address continuing problems—The HFCxA will assist facility staff in developing reports and documents and requests for services to remedy outstanding problems.

6) Lessons learned meeting—The HFCxA will accomplish a meeting with the Owner, contractors, designers, operators, and occupants one year after occupancy to identify lessons learned.

7) Measurement and verification (M&V)

   a) The HFCxA will work with the facility manager to establish a Portfolio Manager account on the EPA Energy Star website.

   b) The HFCxA will help the facility manager enter actual electricity, heating fuel, and water consumption and costs into the Portfolio Manager account.

   c) The HFCxA will assist the facility manager with development of an energy efficiency scorecard and assist the facility manager in publishing the scorecard each month.

   d) If the actual Energy Star rating is less than the target Energy Star rating, the HFCxA will work with the facility manager, design team, and contractor to identify the cause of the disparity and implement corrective action (provide a 40 man-hour contingency for the investigation into why the ES rating is less than the target).

2. WHAT THE COMMISSIONING AUTHORITY IS NOT RESPONSIBLE FOR

The HFCxA is not responsible for design concept, design criteria, compliance with codes, design or general construction scheduling, cost estimating, or construction management. The HFCxA may assist with problem-solving or resolving non-conformance or deficiencies, but ultimately that responsibility resides with the architect and the general contractor.

3. SYSTEMS AND ASSEMBLIES TO BE COMMISSIONED

A. The following systems are to be commissioned:

1) **Building Envelope**

   a) Insulation

   b) Glazing

   c) Vapor barriers

   d) All elements of the building exterior wall

   e) Roof

   f) Building pressure testing

2) **Life Safety**

   a) Fire-resistive ratings

   b) Smoke barriers

   c) Smoke-tight partitions

   d) Stair pressurization system

   e) Fire command center

3) **HVAC Systems**

   a) Air terminals

   b) Induction units

   c) Fan coil units

   d) Unit heaters

   e) Air-handling units

   f) Energy recovery units

   g) Exhaust system

   h) Chilled water system

   i) Heating water system

   j) Steam system

   k) Humidifiers

   l) Fire and smoke dampers

   m) Special applications

   - Operating rooms (anesthetizing locations)
   - Airborne infection isolation (AII) rooms
   - Protective environment (PE) rooms
   - Data center
   - Pharmacy
   - Imaging

4) **Controls**

   a) Workstations

   b) System graphics and dashboards

   c) Networks

   d) Controllers

   e) Sensors

   f) Actuators

   g) Meters

5) **Plumbing Systems**

   a) Domestic cold water

   - Meter
   - Backflow preventers
   - Booster pump
   - Water softener

   b) Domestic hot water

   - Water heater
   - Recirculation system

   c) Sump pumps

   d) Natural gas

   e) Fuel oil

   f) Propane or synthetic natural gas

   g) Disinfection systems

   h) Rainwater harvesting

   i) Process cooling

6) **Medical Gas Systems**

   a) Oxygen

   b) Bulk oxygen system

   c) Remote oxygen supply connection

   d) Nitrogen

e) Nitrous oxide

f) Medical vacuum

g) Waste anesthesia gas disposal

h) Instrument air

i) Medical air

j) Manifold rooms

k) Master and area alarms

l) Valves

- Source
- Future
- Riser
- Service
- Zone

7) **Electrical Systems**

a) Meter

b) Primary transformers

c) Main switchgear

d) Panelboards

e) Isolated power systems

f) Power conditioners

g) Power factor correction equipment

h) Uninterruptible power supplies

i) Step-down transformers

j) Generators

k) Paralleling switchgear

l) Automatic transfer switches

m) Lightning protection systems

n) Grounding systems

8) **Fire Alarm System**

a) Workstations

b) Controllers

c) Sensing devices

d) Interface with life safety systems

e) Interface with fire protection system

f) Interface with HVAC system

g) Interface with elevators

9) **Information Technology**

a) Telephone

b) Data

c) Intercom

d) Paging

e) Doctor's dictation

f) Telemetry

g) Security

h) Master clock

i) Dedicated antenna

j) Television

k) Nurse call

l) Infant abduction

m) Wireless access points

n) Cellular phone repeaters

10) **Fire Protection System**

a) Backflow preventer

b) Fire pump/jockey pump

c) Drains

d) Tamper and flow switches

e) Valves

f) Fire department connections

g) Standpipes

h) Sprinkler heads

i) Pre-action systems

j) Clean agent systems

11) **Interior Lighting**

a) Occupancy sensors

b) Controls

12) Exterior Lighting

a) Controls

b) Illumination levels

13) Refrigeration

a) Food services refrigerators

b) Food services freezers

c) Clinical refrigerators and freezers

d) Blood banks

14) Vertical Transport

a) Elevators

b) Escalators

c) Dumbwaiters

15) Materials and Pharmaceutical Handling

a) Pneumatic tube

b) Linen and trash conveyance

c) Electronic transportation vehicles (ETVs)

4. DESIRED QUALIFICATIONS

A. Principal HFCxA

It is desired that the person designated as the principal HFCxA satisfy the following requirements:

1) Has acted as the principal HFCxA for at least three projects of equivalent or larger size during the past three years.

2) Is experienced in the quality process.

3) Has extensive experience in the operation and troubleshooting of HVAC systems, energy management control systems, and lighting controls systems. Extensive field experience is required. A minimum of five full years in this type of work is required.

4) Is knowledgeable in building operation and maintenance and O&M training.

5) Is knowledgeable in test and balance of both air and water systems.

6) Is experienced in energy-efficient equipment design and control strategy optimization.

7) Has direct experience in monitoring and analyzing system operation using energy management control system trending and stand-alone data logging equipment.

8) Has excellent verbal and written communication skills. Highly organized and able to work with both management and trade contractors.

9) Has a bachelor's degree in Mechanical Engineering and PE certification.

B. HFCxA Team Members

The HFCxA firm will demonstrate depth of experienced personnel and capability to sustain loss of assigned personnel without compromising quality and timeliness of performance.

5. INSTRUCTIONS TO PROPOSERS

A proposer must include execution of all phases of commissioning in a single proposal. The proposal must be signed by an officer of your firm with the authority to commit the firm.

A. Provide a summary description of your firm's commissioning experience within the past five years.

B. Provide a detailed project organizational chart indicating names of dedicated project staff and their specific duties and responsibilities. Provide an organizational chart of your firm.

C. List the key individual who will serve as the principal HFCxA for this contract and describe his or her relevant qualifications and experience. This information is required in addition to any detailed resumes the proposer submits. The contract will require that this individual be committed to the project for its duration.

D. Provide project and professional references and experience for three to five commissioning projects for which the proposer was the principal HFCxA in the last three years. Include a description of each project, identify when the proposer came into the project, and describe the involvement of each individual on the proposer's team in the project. For each project, attach a sheet that includes the name and telephone number of the Owner's project manager.

E. Describe your proposed approach to managing the project expertly and efficiently, including your team participation. Describe what approach you will take to integrate commissioning into the normal design and construction process. Describe what you will do to foster teamwork and cooperation from contractors and designers.

F. As an attachment, provide the following work products written by members of the proposer's team:

1) Commissioning plan that was executed

2) Commissioning specifications

3) An actual Functional Test Procedure that was executed

G. Provide both an estimated total fee to accomplish the work and an hourly rate for each team member. The Owner will negotiate with the selected proposer.

ADDITIONAL CONDITIONS

Owner is not obligated to request clarifications or additional information but may do so at its discretion. Owner reserves the right to extend the deadline for submittals.

Award, if made, shall be to the responsible HFCxA whose proposal is determined in writing to be the most advantageous for the Owner, taking into account all of the evaluation factors set forth in this RFP. No other factors or criteria shall be used in the evaluation. The Owner reserves the right to reject any and all proposals submitted in response to this RFP.

Confidentiality of documents: Upon receipt of a proposal by Owner, the proposal shall become the property of the Owner without compensation to the submitting firm.

RESPONSES ARE DUE (DATE)

Please provide (**xx**) paper copies or one electronic copy (e-mail, CD, or thumb drive media is acceptable).

Sample Commissioning Contract

AGREEMENT FOR COMMISSIONING SERVICES

This Agreement for Commissioning Services ("Agreement") is entered into as of the _____ day of_____, 201__, by and between _____ (the Health Facility Commissioning Authority, hereinafter the "HFCxA"), and _____ (the "Owner").

1. Scope of Work: HFCxA will provide commissioning services with respect to _____ (the "Project") as described in <u>Exhibit A</u> attached hereto. Generally, commissioning is a planned and integrated systematic process to determine, through documented verification, whether all building systems perform interactively according to the design intent. In providing its services, HFCxA will be certifying either (i) that the contractor, subcontractor, architect, designer, engineer, or such other responsible party has demonstrated to HFCxA that the system, equipment, or design was, at the time of certification, functioning in accordance with the plans and specifications of the Project or (ii) that such system, equipment, or design was, at the time of certification, not functioning in accordance with the plans and specifications of the Project.

*However, it is understood and agreed that HFCxA's commissioning services under this Agreement do not include project observation or any other construction phase services that an architect or engineer would usually perform (unless specifically set forth in Exhibit A). Unless Exhibit A provides otherwise, the Owner assumes all responsibility for interpretation of the contract documents and for construction observation and waives any claims against HFCxA that may be in any way connected thereto. HFCxA will assist the Owner as requested and necessary to properly interpret the contract documents to the extent required to successfully complete the commissioning activities and to ensure the owner fully understands the limits and services guarantees in the construction documentation and in the commissioning contracts.

During the Project, HFCxA and Owner may agree to expand HFCxA's scope of services. HFCxA will proceed to provide such additional services five (5) days after it sends to Owner a letter that confirms that the scope of services is to be expanded, describes the additional services to be performed, and sets forth the fee to be charged, unless Owner notifies HFCxA in writing within said five-day period that HFCxA's letter is not accurately set forth by written agreement.

Whether or not HFCxA's scope of services includes project observation or other construction phase services, the parties agree that, during site visits or otherwise, (a) HFCxA shall not be responsible for supervising, inspecting, insuring, warranting, or guaranteeing the means and methods of construction of the Project, (b) HFCxA shall not be responsible for safety at the job site, (c) site visits shall not be relied upon as acceptance of the work, and (d) site visits shall not relieve the Project contractors of their responsibilities and obligations under their respective contracts. HFCxA will make notes of site visit observations and act as the Owner's agent to communicate these observations to the project manager to ensure they become part of the project record and are properly acted on. Appropriate actions include, but may not be limited to, direct communication with the design team or project manager; interactions with the contractor, subcontractor, or other workers found to be engaged in unsafe practices; and communication with the Owner regarding opportunities for improvement in the delivery process.

It is further understood and agreed that HFCxA is not providing a warranty, guarantee, or insurance with respect to any system, equipment, or design. HFCxA does not warrant, guarantee, or insure the systems, equipment, or designs against defects. Further, in providing its services, HFCxA is responsible to validate that systems, equipment, and design are of a particular condition, quality, efficiency, adequacy, or life-expectancy and meet the Owner's Project Requirements.

2. Payment Terms: The Owner agrees to pay HFCxA the amounts set forth in Exhibit A and in any agreement that additional services are to be performed. In addition, Owner agrees to reimburse HFCxA for expenses, including travel, telephone, blueprinting, reproduction, CADD plotting, sales and use taxes, fees required by regulatory agencies for certificates, plan reviews or inspections, express mail, facsimiles, and other postage and shipping charges at actual cost plus a 10 percent (10%) markup for handling. Blueprints and computer-generated plots will be billed for all prints requested by the Owner. The Owner will not be billed for such items used by HFCxA in-house. HFCxA shall provide routine reports on the progress of commissioning activities to the Owner to ensure the Owner has an updated perspective of project progress and expenses related to health facility commissioning activities compared to budget.

HFCxA will bill the Owner monthly with payment to be made within thirty days of invoice date. Interest in the amount of one and one-half percent (1½%) per month shall accrue on all invoices 60 days after invoice date. HFCxA shall have the right to suspend its work on the Project, after giving Owner seven (7) days written notice of its intent to suspend services, if any invoice becomes more than 60 days past due. If the Project is commenced and then for any reason, including but not limited to failure of payment, suspended for more than three months, HFCxA shall have the right to renegotiate the balance of its fee, including increased current Direct Personnel Expense and the cost of project restart, or to terminate this Agreement.

3. Project Completion and Delays: HFCxA is not responsible for delays caused by factors beyond HFCxA's reasonable control, including but not limited to delays because of strikes, lockouts, work slowdowns or stoppages, accidents, and acts of God. When such delays beyond HFCxA's reasonable control occur, or when HFCxA suspends its services due to failure of payment, the Owner agrees that HFCxA is not responsible for damages, nor shall HFCxA be deemed in default of this Agreement. All other delays will be considered a failure of contract and be subject to liquidated damages as specified in Exhibit A.

4. Termination: Either the Owner or HFCxA may terminate this agreement at any time, with or without cause, upon giving the other party fifteen (15) calendar days prior written notice. The Owner shall within thirty (30) calendar days of termination pay HFCxA for all services rendered and all costs incurred up to the date of termination, in accordance with the compensation provisions of this Agreement.

5. Owner's Responsibilities: The Owner shall provide to HFCxA such information about the Project and its design and systems as is available to the Owner and the Owner's consultants and contractors, and HFCxA shall be entitled to rely upon the accuracy and completeness thereof without making independent verification.

The Owner shall obtain the cooperation and assistance of all contractors, subcontractors, architects, designers, and other parties necessary for HFCxA to perform its services, including but not limited to demonstration by such parties that the system, equipment, or design being tested functions in accordance with the plans and specification of the Project and providing any and all materials, records, specification, or other documents as HFCxA may require to perform its services. HFCxA will be responsible for coordinating commissioning activities within the framework of good construction practices consistent with the design team and contractor's schedule. HFCxA is responsible for communicating scheduling problems to the project manager in a timely manner to ensure prompt resolution.

6. Ownership and Use of Reports: In accepting and utilizing any reports or other data generated and provided by HFCxA, the Owner agrees that all such reports and data are instruments of service of HFCxA, who shall be deemed the author of the reports and data and shall retain all common law, statutory and other rights, including copyrights. The Owner further agrees not to use these reports and data, in whole or in part, for any purpose or project other than the Project which is the subject of this Agreement. Reuse of any reports by Owner shall be at Owner's sole risk. HFCxA will make all reports and data collection available to the Owner and the Owner's design team and contractor as necessary for successful and timely project delivery. The overridding determination will be that all data used and collected on the project is the property of the Owner and considered proprietary by the Owner's designation for the purpose of project delivery. Other use of the materials will not be tolerated except as defined by written agreement.

7. Hazardous Materials: It is acknowledged by both parties that HFCxA's scope of services does not include any services related to asbestos or hazardous or toxic materials. In the event HFCxA or any other party encounters asbestos or hazardous or toxic materials at the jobsite, or should it become known in any way that such materials may be present at the jobsite or any adjacent areas that may affect the performance of HFCxA's services, HFCxA may, at its option and without liability for consequential or any other damages, suspend performance of services on the Project until the Owner retains appropriate specialist consultants or contractors to identify, abate and/or remove the asbestos, hazardous or toxic materials and warrant to HFCxA that the jobsite is in full compliance with applicable laws and regulations. HFCxA shall not be responsible in any way for any safety precautions, including measures for the protection of the contractor or any subcontractor, or employees of the Owner, or for the protection of the public.

8. Jobsite Safety: Neither the activities of HFCxA nor the presence of HFCxA at the jobsite shall relieve the Owner, the general contractor, or any other entity of their obligations, duties and responsibilities, including, but not limited to, construction means, methods, sequences, techniques or procedures necessary for performing, superintending or coordinating all portions of the work in accordance with the contract documents and any health or safety precautions required by any regulatory agencies. HFCxA and its personnel have no authority to exercise any control over any construction contractor or other entity or their employees in connection with their work or any health or safety precautions. HFCxA, as an agent for the Owner, will report any safety concerns to the project manager and the Owner to ensure these concerns are documented as part of the project record. HFCxA will provide comments to the Owner regarding opportunities for improvement from observations of coordination activities, sequencing, techniques and procedures, and general project safety.

9. Reliance on Reports: Any report prepared by HFCxA for the Owner is solely and exclusively for Owner's own information and benefit and may not be relied upon by any other person. Owner may, however, distribute copies of such reports to any contractors, subcontractors, architects, designers, or other parties responsible for performance of the Project but such third parties are not intended beneficiaries of this Agreement.

10. Estimates of Probable Cost: To the extent that HFCxA provides the Owner with estimates of the probable cost of work to be performed by others not under the control of HFCxA, Owner understands that HFCxA has no control over costs or the price of labor, equipment or materials, or over the method of pricing. Opinions of probable costs are made on the basis of HFCxA's qualifications and experience. HFCxA makes no warranty, expressed or implied, as to the accuracy of such opinions as compared to actual costs.

11. Damages and Risk Allocation: Notwithstanding any other provision of this Agreement, neither party shall be liable to the other for any consequential damages incurred due to the fault of the other party, regardless of the nature of this fault or whether it was committed by the Owner or HFCxA, their employees, agents, consultants, contractors, subconsultants, or subcontractors.

Consequential damages include, but are not limited to, loss of use and loss of profit. Neither party shall be prevented by this paragraph from recovering expenses or fees associated with the Project.

12. Governing Law: This Agreement shall be construed and interpreted according to the laws of the state of _____.

14. Dispute Resolution: The parties agree to use mediation before litigation in the event a dispute arises that they are not able to resolve themselves. The sole venue for resolution of disputes shall be in _____ (County, State).

15. Entire Agreement: This Agreement and the documents that are expressly incorporated by reference constitute the entire agreement between the parties and supersede all prior and contemporaneous agreements. This Agreement may be modified only in writing signed by both parties.

For HFCxA

_____

Name:
Title:

_____

Date

For (Owner)

_____

Name:
Title:

_____

Date

Sample Owner's Project Requirements for Health Facilities

CONTENTS

INTRODUCTION

The Owner's Project Requirements (OPR) include an introductory section that states the purpose of the OPR. This introductory section should indicate that the primary purpose of the OPR is to document the Owner's goals and requirements for the project. It also indicates that the Owner will develop the OPR at the onset of the project, and the project team will update it periodically to keep it current. This introduction should also indicate that the OPR will be used to measure the success of the project when complete and that all other documents generated during the process (including the Basis of Design, commissioning plan, construction documents, systems manual, etc.) will be compared to the OPR for consistency. Consequently, a comprehensive and accurate OPR is a key element of a successful project.

1. Project Description

The OPR contains a complete description of the project. This should indicate the total building floor area, gross department floor area (GDSF), number of stories, project type (new construction, addition, renovation, etc.), and location.

2. Functional Program

The OPR includes a copy of the functional program for the health care facility. The functional program identifies the services provided by the facility, its departments, anticipated utilization (patient-days, number of visits, etc.), number of employees, and the floor area required for each individual space within each department.

3. Program Flexibility

The OPR indicates which services and departments are most likely to change over time. The OPR identifies special requirements for architectural, structural, mechanical, and electrical system flexibility for these areas. Services and departments that are typically designed for flexibility include food preparation, dining, imaging, and laboratory areas.

4. Future Growth

The OPR indicates which services and departments are most likely to expand over time. The OPR also indicates the minimum amount of equipment, system, and infrastructure spare capacity needed to accommodate future growth. The amount of spare capacity may be as much as 25 percent or more for electrical distribution systems, cooling systems, and heating systems.

5. Longevity

The OPR should indicate the expected useful life of the project. The typical useful life of a health care facility is in the range of 40 to 50 years.

6. Project Cost

The OPR indicates the maximum project cost, inclusive of construction, design fees and expenses, HFCxA fees and expenses, land, utility extension charges, legal fees, hazardous material abatement and disposal (if applicable), medical equipment, furniture, food services equipment, information technology systems, final housekeeping, land costs, legal fees, miscellaneous costs, change order allowance, errors and omissions allowance, and contingencies.

7. Change Orders

The OPR indicates the maximum acceptable change order allowance, which typically is within the range of 1–3 percent of the project budget.

8. Design Errors and Omissions

The OPR indicates the maximum acceptable additional cost resulting from design errors and omissions. The errors and omissions allowance should be in the range of 0.5–1 percent of the project budget.

9. Infection Rates

The OPR indicates maximum acceptable infection rates (MRSA, C-Diff, VRE, etc.) for each department (typically expressed as a percentile ranking).

10. Patient and Visitor Satisfaction

The OPR indicates minimum acceptable patient and visitor satisfaction scores for the facility (typically expressed as a percentile ranking).

11. Appearance

The OPR identifies specific requirements for the exterior appearance of the project, including building elevations, visibility, signage, and landscaping.

The OPR also identifies specific requirements for interior appearance, including finishes, ceiling heights, windows, views, and natural lighting.

12. Maintenance Staffing

The OPR identifies the anticipated maintenance staffing requirement in FTEs or in square feet of floor space per FTE (typically varies from 25,000 to 40,000 SF per FTE for health care facilities). The maintenance staffing requirement is typically determined using the ASHE benchmarking tool.

13. Maintenance Training

The OPR identifies specific training needed for the facility's operations and maintenance staff. The training section should identify the systems and equipment for which training is needed and the preferred training format (classroom, field, etc.).

14. Maintenance Costs

The OPR identifies anticipated maintenance costs for the health care facility, including staffing, service contracts, tools, materials, utilities, and education.

The maintenance cost goal is typically determined using the ASHE benchmarking tool.

15. Operations and Maintenance Dashboards

The OPR identifies the operations and maintenance dashboards to be developed by the project team. These typically include dashboards for building energy demands and costs, major systems, major equipment, and air terminals.

16. Commissioning Tools

The OPR identifies commissioning tools needed by operations and maintenance staff. These tools typically include an open protocol interface to the energy management system and major equipment control panels, an automatic data archiving system, and a query-and-response program.

17. Security

The OPR identifies security requirements for the health care facility. Typical security requirements address building access, secure areas, cameras, emergency phones, and security stations.

18. Thermal Comfort

The OPR identifies thermal comfort goals. Compliance with ANSI/ASHRAE Standard 55: *Thermal Environment Conditions for Human Occupancy* is a typical thermal comfort goal.

19. Regulatory Compliance

The OPR identifies the applicable codes and regulations for the project. Typical codes and regulations applicable to health care facilities are listed below:

- CMS: Health care facilities reimbursed by Medicare or Medicaid are subject to CMS requirements. These requirements include compliance with NFPA 101: *Life Safety Code*.
- Joint Commission: Health care facilities accredited by the Joint Commission are subject to that organization's requirements. These include compliance with all CMS requirements and the Joint Commission's Environment of Care (EC) standards.
- Centers for Disease Control and Prevention (CDC): The CDC *Guidelines for Environmental Infection Control in Health Care Facilities* serves as the basis for many of the Joint Commission's EC standards.
- Occupational Safety and Health Administration (OSHA): OSHA requirements address workplace safety and have a significant impact on the construction and operation of health care facilities.

- U.S. Environmental Protection Agency (EPA): EPA requirements regarding spill prevention from fuel oil tanks, water runoff from construction sites, and air emissions from emergency generators are relevant to the design, construction, and operation of health care facilities.

- United States Pharmacopeia (USP): USP 797 establishes strict requirements for the design and construction of pharmacies where sterile products are prepared.

- Model building codes: A model building code is voluntary unless adopted by state or local legislation. The general purpose of these codes is to regulate the built environment. For more than 50 years, three organizations published model building codes. These organizations published the Uniform Building Code (UBC), Building Officials and Code Administrators (BOCA), and the Southern Building Code (SBC). In general, UBC codes were adopted by western states, BOCA codes were adopted by northeastern states, and SBC codes were adopted by southeastern states. In 1994, UBC, BOCA, and SBC officials founded the International Code Council (ICC). Since then the ICC has published eleven model codes, including a building code, mechanical code, plumbing code, fire code, electrical code, fuel gas code, and energy code. Many states have adopted the ICC code family.

- National fire codes: The National Fire Protection Association (NFPA) publishes a series of fire codes. The NFPA codes most relevant to the planning, design, and construction of health care facilities are as listed here:
  — NFPA 13: *Standard for the Installation of Sprinkler Systems*
  — NFPA 14: *Standard for the Installation of Standpipes and Hose Systems*
  — NFPA 20: *Standard for the Installation of Stationary Pumps for Fire Protection*
  — NFPA 70: *National Electrical Code®*
  — NFPA 90A: *Standard for the Installation of Air-Conditioning and Ventilating Systems*
  — NFPA 90B: *Standard for the Installation of Warm Air Heating and Air-Conditioning Systems*
  — NFPA 96: *Standard for Ventilation Control and Fire Protection of Commercial Cooking Operations*
  — NFPA 99: *Standard for Health Care Facilities*
  — NFPA 101: *Life Safety Code®*
  — NFPA 110: *Standard for Emergency and Standby Power Systems*

- FGI Guidelines: The *Guidelines for Design and Construction of Health Care Facilities* (commonly referred to as the "FGI Guidelines") is published through an agreement between the Facility Guidelines Institute and ASHE. The FGI Guidelines form the basis of more than 40 state health care facility regulations.

- American Society of Heating, Refrigerating and Air-Conditioning Engineers (ASHRAE): ASHRAE publishes a number of documents that are frequently referenced by health care facility codes and regulations. These include those listed below:

  — ASHRAE Standard 15: *Safety Standard for Refrigeration Systems*— This document establishes the minimum requirements for refrigerant machinery rooms.

  — ASHRAE Standards 52.1 and 52.2: These documents establish the testing requirements for determining the dust spot efficiency and minimum efficiency reporting value (MERV) ratings for air filters.

  — ASHRAE Standard 55: *Thermal Environmental Conditions for Human Occupancy*—This document establishes the proper environmental conditions (temperature, humidity, air velocity, etc.) for optimum thermal comfort.

  — ASHRAE Standard 62.1: *Ventilation for Acceptable Indoor Air Quality*—This document establishes minimum ventilation rates and other requirements for many types of buildings including health care facilities.

  — ASHRAE Standard 90.1: *Energy Standard for Buildings Except Low-Rise Residential Buildings*—This document is the basis for many state and local energy codes.

  — ASHRAE Standard 170: *Ventilation of Health Care Facilities*—This document has been incorporated into the 2010 edition of the FGI Guidelines. It establishes standards for HVAC systems, including ventilation rates, pressure relationships, air distribution patterns, design temperatures, design humidity levels, and infection control procedures.

- State regulations: State regulation of health care facilities is typically multi-faceted, involving numerous agencies and regulations. In general, however, state regulations include the following:

  — Building and fire codes: Most states have adopted a specific edition of the ICC codes or one of the other model building codes with state-specific amendments as their building and fire code. Building and fire codes establish specific requirements based on type of occupancy, type of construction, and other parameters. In many states, building and fire code enforcement is provided by city inspectors under the jurisdiction of local fire departments or a state fire marshal.

— Mechanical code: Most states have adopted a specific edition of the *International Mechanical Code*® or one of the other model building codes. In many states, mechanical code enforcement is provided by city inspectors under the jurisdiction of a contractor's licensing board.

— Electrical code: Most states have adopted a specific edition of NFPA 70: *National Electrical Code*®. In most states, city inspectors enforce the electrical code.

— Boiler code: Most states have adopted a boiler code. The boiler code addresses the installation, operation, attendance, and maintenance of boilers and other pressure vessels. In most states, boiler code enforcement is provided by a state agency.

— Gas code: Most states have adopted a specific edition of the *International Fuel Gas Code*®. In most states, gas code enforcement is provided by city inspectors under the jurisdiction of a state agency.

— Energy code: Most states have adopted either ASHRAE 90.1 or a specific edition of the *International Energy Conservation Code*®. In most states, city officials under the jurisdiction of a state agency enforce the energy code.

— Food services: Most states have adopted regulations for food preparation and serving facilities. In most states, enforcement is provided by local inspectors under the jurisdiction of a state agency.

— Elevators: Many states have adopted specific requirements for the construction of elevator hoistways and machine rooms. These requirements frequently address fire-resistive ratings, fire protection systems, fire alarm systems, and the elevator electrical service (shunt trip). In most states, enforcement of elevator regulations is provided by a state agency.

— Pharmacy: Many state pharmacy boards have adopted USP 797.

— Medical waste: Many states have adopted specific regulations concerning the storage, transportation, and disposal of medical waste.

— Environmental quality: Most states have agencies responsible for the enforcement of EPA regulations. Although similar, these state regulations frequently vary from the federal requirements. These requirements address air emissions from boilers and emergency generators.

— Health department: Most states have adopted regulations based on a specific edition of the FGI *Guidelines for Design and Construction of Health Care Facilities*. It is not uncommon, however, for the state regulations to include amendments or variations from the FGI Guidelines.

- Local regulations: Many cities and counties have adopted local codes and regulations, which may vary from state and federal codes. Several cities have adopted sustainability requirements and often require LEED certification.

The OPR also addresses building occupancy and project type. Most codes and regulations are based on building occupancy. Building occupancy types include Assembly, Residential, Institutional, Business, and others. In general, hospitals are considered Institutional occupancies. Certain areas within the hospital, however, may be separated from the Institutional occupancy and considered to be Assembly or Business occupancies. Establishing the building occupancy is typically the first step of a project-specific code search.

The codes and regulations that may be applicable to a specific project also depend on the type of project. In general, codes and regulations are more stringent for new construction projects. A partial listing of project types is provided here:

- New construction: Most codes and regulations are intended for new construction. New construction would include additions to existing facilities and new facilities. A new construction hospital project would be required to comply with Chapter 18 of the *Life Safety Code*, which mandates the installation of automatic sprinklers.

- Major renovation: A major renovation is typically defined as a modification of more than 50 percent of a smoke compartment or 4,500 square feet of a smoke compartment. Major renovations are typically subject to the requirements for new construction.

- Minor renovation: A minor renovation is typically defined as a modification that is not large enough to be considered a major renovation (see statistics in paragraph above). Minor renovations are typically subject to code requirements for existing facilities. A minor renovation hospital project would be required to comply with Chapter 19 of the *Life Safety Code*, which does not mandate installation of automatic sprinklers.

- Maintenance and repair: Many regulations provide allowances for maintenance and repair projects. The repair or replacement of existing equipment with similar equipment is usually not subject to current codes provided the existing level of life safety is not diminished. Many codes also provide allowances for projects that are implemented in phases (e.g., entire systems are generally not required to be upgraded to current codes during the first phase of the work).

20. SYSTEM RELIABILITY

The OPR identifies specific requirements for equipment and system reliability. The reliability requirements for a health care facility may include those listed below:

- N plus 1 reliability for emergency power, cooling, and heating systems
- Multiple fans in air handling units serving critical areas
- 100% generator capacity (entire facility can be served from the generators)
- Paralleling switchgear with load shedding capability
- On-site Fuel Storage
- Dual fuel capability

21. PROJECT SCHEDULE

The OPR establishes the target completion date for the project. If the project involves multiple phases, the OPR should establish the target completion date for each phase.

22. SUSTAINABILITY

The OPR establishes the project sustainability goals. The typical sustainability rating systems for health care facilities are listed here:

- Leadership in Energy and Environmental Design (LEED®): The LEED rating system for sustainable design is administered by the U.S. Green Building Council (USGBC). There are various levels of LEED certification, including certified, silver, gold, and platinum. The USGBC is developing a sustainability rating system specifically for health care facilities (LEED for Health Care).
- Green Guidelines for Healthcare Facilities (GGHC): GGHC is a self-administered rating system similar to the LEED process, but it also includes operational issues.
- ASHRAE Standard 189.2: ASHRAE has proposed a new standard that will address the design, construction, and operation of high performance health care facilities.

23. ENERGY EFFICIENCY

The OPR establishes the project energy efficiency goal, typically expressed as a target Energy Star rating. For new facilities, the recommended Energy Star target rating is 75 (the minimum required to earn the Energy Star label). For renovation and building addition projects, the recommended Energy Star target rating should be a reasonable increase from the current and baseline energy ratings for the existing facility.

24. QUALITY OF BUILDING MATERIALS AND FINISHES

The OPR establishes the desired quality of building materials and finishes. The OPR addresses longevity, cleaning requirements, supplier locations, and minimum inventories.

25. BUILDING MAINTENANCE PROGRAM

The OPR addresses requirements for the development and implementation of a building maintenance program (BMP). The BMP typically utilizes a computerized maintenance management system (CMMS). The BMP should include a work order system for scheduled and unscheduled equipment and system maintenance. The OPR should also stipulate additional BMP requirements, such as those listed here:

- Ensure that all equipment is numbered and labeled in a manner consistent with facility standards. For renovation and addition projects, the equipment numbers should begin with the next available number (not start over again at 1).

- Ensure that room numbers indicated on the construction drawings are consistent with facility standards and actual room numbers. The actual room numbers are frequently different from the room numbers indicated on the construction drawings; this inconsistency creates difficulty for the O&M staff and poses a significant barrier to achieving an effective transition from construction completion to sustainable operation.

- Ensure the Owner receives an electronic archive of all information required to operate and maintain the facility.

- Ensure each item of equipment and its associated maintenance and operating information are identified in the CMMS.

- Ensure the CMMS automatically generates work orders for recommended maintenance procedures at the recommended frequency.

- Ensure a complete service history for each item of equipment (scheduled maintenance, unscheduled maintenance, etc.) is maintained in the CMMS.

- Ensure the CMMS provides for regular (annual or more frequent) calibration of temperature, pressure, and other sensors critical to efficient system performance.

26. UTILITY MANAGEMENT PLAN

The OPR identifies specific requirements for the Utility Management Plan (UMP). The UMP is required by the Joint Commission's *2010 Comprehensive Accreditation Manual for Hospitals* and should include the following sections:

- Written inventories of the operating components of utility systems considered critical to patient care based on risks of infection and occupant needs
- Written descriptions of inspection, testing, and maintenance activities for operating components of critical utility systems
- Detailed diagrams of utility distribution systems
- Written procedures for responding to utility system disruptions
- Written procedures for shutting off malfunctioning utility systems and notifying staff in affected areas
- Written procedures for obtaining emergency repair services
- Written identification of alternative means of providing electricity, water, and fuel
- Written identification of alternative means for providing medical air, medical vacuum, oxygen, nitrous oxide, nitrogen, and other medical gases
- Written identification of alternative means of providing other critical utilities, such as vertical transport, steam for sterilization, heating, cooling, and ventilation
- Written procedures for responding to events that curtail or disrupt utility service to the health care facility for up to 96 hours

27. FIRE AND SMOKE DAMPER TESTING

The OPR identifies requirements for fire and smoke damper testing. National codes require health care facilities to inspect and test their fire and smoke dampers within 12 months of installation and every six years thereafter. To reduce costs and minimize disruption, the initial damper inspection and testing should occur immediately prior to occupancy.

28. SYSTEMS MANUAL

The OPR identifies the requirements for a systems manual. At a minimum, this manual should include the final versions of the OPR and the BOD, system single-line drawings, as-built sequences of operation, control shop drawings, original control set points, operating instructions for integrated systems, recommended retesting schedules and blank test forms, sensor and actuator recalibration schedules, and a condensed troubleshooting guide for operations and maintenance personnel.

29. WARRANTY PERIOD

The OPR indicates the expected warranty period. The typical warranty period for new construction and renovation projects is one year from the date of substantial completion. The warranty typically covers defects in equipment, materials, and workmanship.

30. PREFERRED MANUFACTURERS

The OPR indicates preferred manufacturers for equipment and systems, including water chillers, cooling towers, air-handling units, boilers, pumps, generators, switchgears, controls system, and fire alarm system.

31. OUTDOOR AND INDOOR DESIGN CONDITIONS

The OPR indicates the outdoor and indoor design conditions. The outdoor design conditions are typically expressed as follows:

- Peak cooling airflow requirements shall be calculated using the ASHRAE 0.4% dry bulb temperature and the mean coincident wet bulb temperature.
- Peak cooling refrigeration (tons) and chilled water flow (GPM) requirements shall be calculated using the ASHRAE 0.4% wet bulb temperature, mean coincident dry bulb temperature, and the peak cooling airflow requirements.
- Peak heating requirements shall be calculated using the ASHRAE 99.6% dry bulb temperature.
- Peak humidification requirements shall be calculated using the ASHRAE 99.6% dry bulb temperature and the mean coincident wet bulb temperature.

The indoor design conditions should comply with the minimum standards of the FGI Guidelines. The interior design conditions are typically expressed as follows:

- Office and administrative
    - Cooling—72 deg. F and 60% RH
    - Heating—70 deg. F
- Classrooms
    - Cooling – 75 deg. F and 55% RH
    - Heating—68 deg. F
- Laboratories
    - Cooling—72 deg F and 60% RH
    - Heating—70 deg. F and 35% RH
- Corridors
    - Cooling—75 deg. F and 55% RH
    - Heating—68 deg. F
- Lobbies
    - Cooling—75 deg. F and 55% RH
    - Heating—68 deg. F
- Mechanical rooms
    - Cooling—90 deg. F
    - Heating—60 deg. F
- Electrical rooms
    - Cooling—80 deg. F
    - Heating—60 deg. F
- Telephone/data rooms
    - Cooling—68 deg. F and 60% RH
    - Heating—68 deg. F
- Public toilet rooms
    - Cooling—75 deg. F and 55% RH
    - Heating—68 deg. F
- Data centers
    - Cooling—70 deg. F and 60% RH
    - Heating—68 deg. F and 40% RH

- Patient rooms and airborne infection isolation rooms
  — Cooling—72 deg. F and 60% RH
  — Heating—70 deg. F
- Exam rooms, treatment rooms, and triage rooms
  — Cooling—72 deg. F and 60% RH
  — Heating—70 deg. F
- Operating rooms, trauma rooms, special procedures rooms, and cath labs
  — Cooling—62 deg. F and 55% RH
  — Heating—75 deg. F and 35% RH

32. MEASUREMENT AND VERIFICATION OF ENERGY EFFICIENCY

The OPR identifies the requirements for measuring and verifying actual building energy performance using the Energy Star rating system. If the actual Energy Star rating does not meet or exceed the target rating, the project team should work to identify the cause of the disparity and implement corrective action.

33. JOINT COMMISSION STATEMENT OF CONDITIONS

The OPR identifies the requirements for completing the Joint Commission Statement of Conditions (SOC), if applicable. The project team should complete the SOC immediately prior to occupancy.

34. GUIDE FOR CONSULTANTS AND CONTRACTORS

The OPR includes compliance requirements for the "Owner's Guide for Consultants and Contractors," where applicable. The guide typically identifies mandatory requirements for materials, workmanship, equipment, and systems.

35. ASHE CERTIFICATES AND CERTIFICATIONS

The OPR indicates ASHE certification requirements for project team members. Recommended requirements are as follows:

- Health Care Project Management Certificate (HCPM)—Project manager, facility manager, architect, engineer, and construction manager
- Certified Health Care Constructor (CHC) certification—Construction manager, general contractor, mechanical subcontractor, and electrical subcontractor

- Health Care Construction Certificate (HCC)—Construction manager, general contractor, mechanical subcontractor, and electrical subcontractor
- Infection Control Certificate (ICC)—Project manager, facility manager, architect, engineer, construction manager, and general contractor

36. EXTENDED WARRANTIES

The OPR indicates requirements for extended warranties on major equipment such as water chillers, cooling towers, boilers, generators, and switchgear.

37. CONSTRUCTION DOCUMENTS

The OPR indicates requirements for the construction documents format. Current best practice is to use building information modeling (BIM) software to create a building information model, which can be used during design, construction, and operation of the health care facility.

38. CLOSEOUT DOCUMENTS

The OPR indicates requirements for closeout documents, including TAB reports, electrical tests, fire alarm tests, maintenance manuals, and record drawings.

39. PROJECT DELIVERY METHOD

The OPR indicates the selected project delivery method. Typical project delivery methods for health care projects include design-bid-build, construction manager-at-risk, and design-build.

40. MEDICAL ERRORS

The OPR indicates the maximum acceptable medical error rate (typically expressed as a percentile rating).

41. CONSTRUCTION RISK ASSESSMENT

If the project is a renovation or addition, the OPR indicates the construction risk assessment requirements. Part of the construction risk assessment is an infection control risk assessment (ICRA). The ICRA is a tool used to determine the potential risk of causing the spread of infection during construction, renovation, and maintenance activities. Based on the results of the assessment, control measures are put into place that reduce this risk.

42. INTERIM LIFE SAFETY MEASURES

If the project is a renovation or addition, the OPR indicates the life safety features that will be affected by the project and the interim life safety measures (ILSMs) to be employed to mitigate safety risks.

43. UTILITY AND EQUIPMENT SHUTDOWNS

If the project is a renovation or addition, the OPR indicates measures to be taken to minimize utility and equipment shutdowns as well as the notice requirements for utility and equipment shutdowns that cannot be avoided.

44. ACOUSTICS

The OPR indicates the acoustic requirements for the project. These are typically expressed in the form of room criteria (RC) as indicated below. Also see Table 1.2-2: Minimum–Maximum Design Criteria for Noise in Interior Spaces in the 2010 FGI *Guidelines for Design and Construction of Health Care Facilities.*

Type of Room/Space	Recommended RC Level
Type	RC Curve
Patient rooms	30–40 (N)
Operating rooms	35–45 (N)*
Laboratories	40–50 (N)
Corridors	35–45 (N)
Public areas	35–45 (N)

*See A1.2-6.1.4 in the 2010 Guidelines for a caveat regarding achieving this sound level in operating rooms.

45. BUILDING PRESSURE TESTING

The OPR indicates requirements for building pressure testing, which should confirm that the building envelope is properly sealed.

46. ROOM PRESSURE TESTING

The OPR indicates requirements for room pressure testing, which should confirm that rooms required to have either positive or negative pressure relationships are properly sealed.

Sample Basis of Design Document

BASIS OF DESIGN DOCUMENT FOR SUSTAINABLE DESIGN AND CONSTRUCTION

Overview

(Client Name) has been designed to perform as a top-of-the-line hospital, with patient care and green principles guiding building function and form. The building envelope, HVAC systems, plumbing system, electrical systems, and other building components have been designed to meet the owner's wishes and the program requirements for the project. This building will be outfitted with a digital electronic-controlled building automation system (BAS) that will receive feedback regarding several parameters, including ventilation, humidity, and temperature. The building envelope and MEP systems are designed in accordance with several standards and criteria, including:

- Energy performance per ASHRAE 90.1-2004
- CFC-free HVAC equipment
- Compliance with ASHRAE 62.1-2001
- Thermal comfort parameters in accordance with ASHRAE 55-2004
- Water savings above the standards set by the Energy Policy Act of 1992

General Design Conditions

Space Use, Diversity, and Space Environmental Requirements

The replacement facility for (Client Name) is a 616,750-square-foot design on a 42.8-acre setting. The use of the building will be typical of a hospital and will include the following:

- Inpatient and outpatient services
- General practice
- Acute care
- Surgical operations
- Regular visitation

As such, different areas of the hospital will require varied amounts of environmental control regulated by an automated control system for the efficiency and sustainability of the delicate, sterile environment.

Occupancy

The hospital is estimated to have a full-time equivalent (FTE) occupancy of 1,552 and a part-time equivalent (PTE) occupancy of 1,387 (304 visitors/day and 1,083 outpatients/day).

Climatic Design Conditions

The building's location in (Facility Location) is designated Climate Zone 4A. The following table shows the climatic conditions used for building load and comfort calculations.

Weather Data	
Latitude (Degrees)	
Longitude (Degrees)	
Summer Design DB/WB (°F)	93/75
Winter Design DB/WB (°F)	12/NA

Building Envelope

The building exterior will primarily be composed of a brick façade, glazed curtain wall assemblies, and stone veneer. Vision and spandrel glazing will be part of the pre-finished aluminum curtain wall system, which will be banded with stone veneer at each floor level. The curtain wall will comprise the aluminum structure and 1" insulated glass that is backed by a 2" airspace, rigid insulation, fibrous insulation in a metal stud cavity, and gypsum board. A significant area of the exterior will be exposed brick. Sections of the building will also be built with a stone veneer. The typical building section for the brick wall areas will include the brick, a 2" airspace, a 6" insulation cavity, and ⅝" drywall on the interior of the building. The typical roof section comprises a high SRI roofing product of either a TPO membrane or an SBS Bitumen product. This material will be on a substrate of approximately 3" of tapered, insulated lightweight concrete on top of 3+ inches of rigid foam insulation.

HVAC&R

Chilled Water System

The chilled water system will include three 800-ton centrifugal water-cooled chillers, Trane CVHF, to serve the entire new facility. Two chillers will be required to meet peak demand load, with one chiller always available in standby mode or to allow chiller maintenance. One of the two operating chillers will have a VFD. A fourth chiller has been included in the plans for future expansion. All chilled water systems shall be based on zero use of CFC-based refrigerants.

Chilled water distribution will be variable primary. The chillers will be served by four chilled water variable flow pumps with three pumps distributing 42°F supply water and one pump standby (16° Delta-T on chilled water system, 2000 GPM per pump). Pumps will be controlled by Tek Works chiller plant optimization controls. The primary piping loop within the chiller room will be constructed with 18" diameter schedule 40 steel piping. 18" chilled water supply and return mains shall be routed through Access corridor to the hospital/MOB.

The condenser water system will consist of one pump per chiller (2,400 GPM each) serving four 2-cell, 800-ton, induced draft cooling towers. The cooling towers will be located on the roof of the Central Energy Plant (CEP) and shall be equal to Marley NC8305H (6,400 ton cells, 78°F WB ambient, 85–95°F water operating range), stainless steel, with 30 hp fan and VFD per cell. Electric basin heaters will provide freeze protection for the basin in the winter time.

Steam and Heating Water Systems

Three 500 BHP steam boilers will serve the entire facility. A fourth boiler is planned for any future expansion. Two boilers will be required to meet peak demand load with one boiler always available in standby mode to allow boiler maintenance. Boilers will be firetube, wetback design, dual fuel (natural gas and No. 2 fuel oil), equipped with 30 ppm low NOX burners and shall be Cleaver Brooks 4WI. One boiler will have a tri-fuel burner to burn landfill gas from a nearby county landfill. Flue gas economizers will recover heat from the boiler stacks and reheat the heating hot water returns. A vortex shedding flow-meter in the steam main will record instantaneous header pressure and steam flow and connect to building automation system for monitoring purposes. Boiler controls will be integrated with DDC control systems to monitor critical boiler functions.

A deaerator (0.005 cc/liter), Industrial Steam Spray Flow II Model 15SP5II or equal, shall collect/treat steam condensate and provide boiler feedwater to each of the boilers. The deaerator will have two recycle pumps and three boiler feedwater pumps (one future pump will be added with expansion). A boiler chemical feed system will be provided. All feedwater pumps shall be piped into common header and controls shall start a feedwater pump for each boiler that is operational. Boiler feedwater pumps shall run continuously when a boiler is placed in operation (modulating feedwater makeup). Deaerator shall come complete with factory-mounted controls, motor starters, pump on, pump off, pump alarm indicating lights, water level controls, high and low water level alarms and contacts for interfacing with building automation system. Deaerator shall also be factory equipped with sample cooler.

Medium pressure steam (80 psi) will be routed from the CEP (10") to hot water room in the main building. Steam piping will be schedule 40 black steel and condensate piping will be schedule 80 black steel. A steam pressure reducing station in hot water room (within the building) will reduce pressure from 80 to 30 psig to serve kitchen appliances, domestic water heaters, building heating heat exchangers and humidifiers. Provide two pressure regulating valves in parallel. Low pressure steam will be distributed to steam/hot water heat exchangers in each location sized as follows:

Ground floor (hot water room):	18,000 MBH
North ground-level mechanical room (serves inpatient):	18,300 MBH
North ground-level mechanical room (serves outpatient):	1,950 MBH
OR penthouse unit (serves ORs and interventional labs):	3,300 MBH

Duplex condensate receiver/pump sets (refer to attached equipment forms) will be at each location to collect and pump condensate back to the central plant. High pressure steam and medium pressure steam will be piped to respective sterilizers and humidifier loads at designated air-handling units (refer to attached equipment forms).

Heating water piping systems from the above-indicated heat exchangers will include two pumps per system, one standby. Heating water piping will be routed to terminal reheat boxes, unit heater in penthouses and cabinet unit heaters in entrance vestibules and stair towers.

Air Distribution Systems

The hospital will be served by approximately 24 indoor chilled water air-handling units (see attached air-handling sheets). Fan coil units will serve stair # 4 and stair # 1, hot water room, elevator machine rooms, loading dock, meeting rooms, outside air and exit passageway (1503, 1405A). The central station units will provide conditioned air via medium/high pressure ductwork to hot water terminal reheat boxes (constant or variable volume, depending upon space served). These boxes will temper the air as necessary to control space temperature and supply air will then be distributed via low pressure duct to the outlets. Return air will be ducted back to the return fans. Air from soiled and contaminated spaces will be mechanically exhausted by fans located within penthouses or roof mounted. Air terminal boxes will be provided on the return air at selected spaces for pressure control. All air distribution systems shall be based on zero use of CFC-based refrigerants.

Special requirements for the air distribution system shall include the following: Pharmacy and Lab hood ductwork (approximately five hoods) shall be 18-gauge welded stainless steel and shall be routed to roof-mounted exhaust fans. The kitchen hood exhaust ductwork will be routed to a roof-mounted fan and will be welded black steel. The dishwasher hood ductwork will be welded aluminum. Central sterile exhaust systems shall be 18-gauge welded stainless steel. MRI ductwork shall be aluminum. Supply air diffusers serving operating rooms, C-section rooms, trauma rooms, and interventional labs shall be two foot by four foot laminar flow diffusers with integral HEPA filters.

Each central AHU system shall consist of an air-handling unit (AHU) with a chilled water coil, preheat coil (selected units only), stand-alone return air fan, 100% airside economizer, and 95% efficient filters downstream of supply fans. Airflow measurement stations will be provided on the supply and return ductwork to AHUs. These stations will verify minimum quantities of outdoor air are provided via synchronized volumetric tracking. Preheat coils shall be served by in-line hot water recirculating freeze protection pumps in the preheat coil piping. Both supply and return fan motors shall be served by VFDs, except for units in CEP and kitchen makeup air units. Each air-handling unit will have sound attenuators located at supply and return duct connections to reduce sound levels (Vibro Acoustics or equivalent).

Provide sound attenuators on exhaust fans and air terminal units as required by attenuator manufacturer calculations to meet required sound levels. The A/C units shall be zoned as follows:

ACU	Zone Served	CFM	Location	Type
1	Plan East Tower floors 5–1	61,500	Plan East Tower penthouse	Custom penthouse
2	Plan North Tower floors 5–2	81,600	Plan North Tower penthouse	Custom penthouse
3	Plan West Tower floors 5–2	81,600	Plan West Tower penthouse	Custom penthouse
4	Plan South Tower floors 5–1	61,500	Plan South Tower penthouse	Custom penthouse
5	Patient Tower core fl. 2–5	47,000	Core Tower penthouse – 6th floor	Semi-custom
6	Inpatient surgery/2nd floor	41,000	2nd floor penthouse	Custom penthouse
7	Surgery/2nd floor	21,000	2nd floor penthouse	Custom penthouse
8	Surgery/OA unit	23,500	2nd floor penthouse	Custom penthouse
9	1st Emergency department	27,500	1st floor mechanical room	Semi-custom
10	1st Emergency department - 2	36,160	1st floor mechanical room	Semi-custom
11	1st Imaging	32,700	Ground level mech. room	Semi-custom
12	Ground level lab	21,500	Ground level mech. room	Semi-custom
13	1st Cardio suite	43,100	Ground level mech. room	Semi-custom
14	ASC – Level 1	16,300	Ground level mech. room	Semi-custom
15	ASC – Level 2	29,600	Ground level mech. room	Semi-custom
16	Lower level CS	16,200	Ground level mech. room	Semi-custom
17	Lower level garden	60,300	Ground level mech. room	Semi-custom
18	Lobby 2-1	42,000	Ground level mech. room	Semi-custom
19	Lower level	25,000	Ground level mech. room	Modular
20	Lower dining level kitchen	23,000	Ground Level mech. room	Modular
21	Kitchen makeup unit	4,500	Ground level mech. room	Modular
22	CEP – Chiller	12,000	CEP	Modular
23	CEP – Electrical rooms	8,000	CEP	Modular
24	CEP – Shop/medical gas/fire pump	4,200	CEP	Modular

All custom patient tower AHUs shall have dual supply fans each with their own VFD.

Operating/Interventional Lab/C-section rooms/trauma rooms: Each room will be served by a dedicated digital electronic, independent pressure variable air volume (VAV) box with hot water reheat coil. In addition, each room shall have a dedicated digital electronic, independent pressure variable air volume (VAV) box located in the return duct to maintain each room except for trauma rooms) at a positive pressure regardless of whether room is occupied or unoccupied. Each room will be provided with a digital electronic control panel that displays both room actual temperature and humidity and also displays both temperature and humidity setpoints. Each room will be provided with room occupancy sensors that will be utilized in determining whether room is "occupied" or "unoccupied." When space is "unoccupied" both supply and return airflow will be reduced by two-thirds of the "occupied" airflow. Each room shall also be equipped with a differential pressure room monitor with connection to the building automation system (BAS).

Provide a low-temp coil for outside air AHU (AHU-8) serving operating room (ACU-6,7) to maintain space at 65 degrees F and 50–60% relative humidity. OA unit shall have two coils: one standard chilled water coil and one low-temp glycol coil. Provide a 125-nominal-ton water-cooled glycol chiller and two 300 gpm pumps at 160 feet of head to serve low-temp coil. All low-temp equipment shall be located in CEP.

For operating room AHU provide smoke evacuation control sequence to vent smoke in accordance with NEPA 99. Smoke evacuation shall be accomplished by relieving 100% of return air.

Specialty Air Conditioning

MRI computer equipment rooms will have 8-ton ceiling-mounted computer room split system. These split systems will have glycol-cooled condensing units. Air conditioning unit for computer equipment rooms will be complete with DDC controls, hot water reheat coil, and steam humidifier. The glycol-cooled condensing units will be mounted above the ceiling with the drycooler located outside, at grade. All specialty air conditioning systems shall be based on zero use of CFC-based refrigerants.

Magnetic resonance imaging rooms: MRI room will be served by a dedicated digital electronic, independent pressure variable air volume (VAV) box with hot water reheat coil. MRI room shall also be equipped with an oxygen deficiency monitor with connection to the building automation system (BAS). Under normal operation air supplied to the room will be returned to the air-handling system. However, in the event of cryogen release (as detected by the oxygen deficiency monitor), a dedicated fan will be energized and air from the room will be exhausted to the outdoors. Dampers in the return air duct will prevent oxygen deficient air from being returned to the air-handling system.

Process air-cooled chillers for the MRI and CT Room equipment cooling will be provided by the imaging equipment vendor.

Laboratory: The laboratory will be served by air terminal boxes on supply and exhaust ducts to maintain the laboratory at a constant negative pressure relative to adjacent areas. Laboratory areas will be served by hot water reheat coils and wall-mounted temperature transmitters monitored through the building automation system. The laboratory will also be equipped with a differential pressure room monitor with connection to the building automation system (BAS).

Ventilation Systems

General exhaust fans: Provide general exhaust fans that are dedicated and interlocked with their respective air-handling unit. Fans will be of the belt driven utility set or PRE type.

Isolation room exhaust fans: Provide fan systems for serving multiple stacked isolation rooms. Each isolation room will be served by dedicated air terminal boxes for modulating supply/exhaust airflows as required to maintain differential offset between supply and exhaust. Each room shall also be served by dedicated hot water reheat coil and wall-mounted temperature transmitter through the building automation system (BAS). Each room shall also be equipped with a differential pressure room monitor with connection to the BAS. Each exhaust fan will be served by a HEPA filter bank module located upstream of the exhaust fan inlet. Each fan will be equipped with a variable frequency drive and duct static pressure transducer upstream of filter bank to maintain a constant duct static pressure regardless of filter loading.

Fuel Oil Systems

One belowground fiberglass, double-wall fuel oil tank at 25,000 gallons will provide No. 2 fuel oil (diesel) to the boilers and emergency generators. A second 30,000 gallon tank will be added as an additional alternate. Duplex fuel oil pump sets (one pump redundant) with 40 GPM fuel oil at 50 psig. will be mounted on the fuel oil tanks. Fuel oil pump controls shall be by building automation system for the generators, and manual switchover for the boilers. Fuel oil pump sets shall be piped to all generators and boilers in pressurized loop for each system with backpressure valve for each loop. Individual solenoid valves and pressure reducing valves will provide fuel oil to generator day tanks based on level control switches mounted in generator day tanks.

Fuel oil monitoring and inventory system as manufactured by Veeder-Root or equal will monitor the entire fuel oil system and connect to the BAS for alarm reporting.

HVAC Control System

A facility wide digital electronic building automation system (BAS) will be installed. All mechanical equipment will be connected and controlled/monitored by the BAS. All equipment items shall be mapped to graphical screens that are provided on the front end computer workstation to be located in the engineering department of this facility.

Provide 10 HP duplex reciprocating air compressor as required to provide control air for the operation of pneumatic actuators serving large control valves and large dampers located in central energy plant pneumatic valves located in the laboratory for the BSL-3 area.

Two operator workstations with full graphic system representation shall be provided to provide control and monitoring capabilities.

Control wiring shall be in conduit and shall be installed to meet Division 16 requirements.

Flow meters will be provided in the steam piping and a flow/BTU meter in chilled water leaving the CEP so the usage of these services can be tracked by percentage basis. All meters will be monitored by the hospital's control system and provided by Onicon or equal.

A CO_2-based monitoring system will control space ventilation for high-occupancy spaces per ASHRAE 62-2001.

Smoke Control/High-Rise Considerations

Stairwell pressurization will be provided for stairwells above 75 feet above the basement level. These stairwells will be provided with sidewall supply grilles to pressurize the stairwell. Selective stairwell doors (approximately four per stair) will be provided with differential pressure monitors to control stairwell pressurization fans. Stairwell pressurization fans shall be centrifugal roof-mounted fans (approximately 16,000 cfm). A relief penthouse with counterbalanced damper shall be provided at the top of stair for required relief. Smoke detectors shall be provided in the duct inlets to the pressurization fans along with smoke dampers.

Exhaust fans are provided in the atrium ceiling to exhaust per the *International Building Code* for atriums. These fans will exhaust approximately 101,000 cfm (33,760 cfm per fan) from the atrium.

Service Water Heating

Domestic Water Systems

The new facility will be served from the local utilities provided by the civil engineer to the building.

Domestic cold water will consist of an 8″ water main routed into the central energy plant. The incoming supply will be routed through two 8″ reduced pressure backflow preventers prior to entering a triplex booster pump system. All water will be boosted to 80 psig discharge leaving the booster pump. The supply will then be routed through a duplex water softener system to reduce the total hardness to zero grains water hardness. As the water leaves this unit it will be manually blended to achieve 3 to 5 GPG water hardness before continuing. A separate duplex boiler softener will be used to provide zero grains water hardness to the boiler make-up and quick fill connections on this equipment.

Domestic hot water will be provided from two 120° and two 140° semi-instantaneous steam-fired water heaters.

Both systems will be 100% redundancy in capacity. Both will contain hot water recirculation piped systems with balancing valves at all branches. Pumps will be provided in the CEP as well as at remote areas to maintain water temperatures throughout the system. System piping will be copper with all piping over 4″ in size having brazed joints.

The restrooms in the building will be outfitted with water-conserving fixtures to save water above the standards set by the Energy Policy Act of 1992. Patient and staff restrooms will include water closets with dual flush handles, allowing for a flush of 1.1 GPF, and low-flow lavatories with flow rates of 2 GPM. Public restrooms will be outfitted with very low-flow lavatories with flow rates of 1 GPM and photo-eye sensors set at 12 seconds.

Power

Utility Service

Baseline utility service from (Electrical Provider) will consist of two (2) underground 25kV feeders brought to the campus from two different substations. The two feeders will be terminated in a pad mount, non-automatic selector switch on the campus property that will serve as the origin point for a 25kV primary distribution loop. The campus will receive service from (Electrical Provider) at 25kV (primary metering) by way of a primary distribution loop. The design of the loop and the associated primary distribution equipment (sectionalizer switches, vacuum breakers, transformers, etc.) will be by (Electrical Provider). Each building will tap off of the loop and receive service at 480V, by way of pad-mounted transformers, as described in the sections that follow.

To reduce demand charges from the utility, the hospital has negotiated a Load Control Rate with (Electrical Provider) to reduce their coincident peak demand charges to zero. Under this scenario (Electrical Provider) will send coincident peak signals to the hospital (assuming 100% liability if they fail to do so) notifying them of an upcoming peak. At that point, the hospital will start their stand-by generators and run in parallel with the utility until the peak has passed. (Electrical Provider) anticipates 150 to 200 hours of load control per year. No reverse power flow will be permitted.

To achieve the Load Control Rate, the hospital will install a 100% standby power system that will be designed for parallel connection to the (Electrical Provider) grid. In this manner, (Client) will be able to drop to 0kW demand during utility coincident peak hours. (Client) currently owns a 2000 kW (1825 kW prime) diesel generator that will be relocated to the site (adjacent to the MOB) and tied into the (Electrical Provider) grid by way of a 3000 kVA, 480Y/277:25kV, pad-mounted, oil-filled transformer (by (Electrical Provider)). This generator will serve as the legally required essential system power source, as well as the prime power source in the Load Control Rate mode for the MOB. The generator output will tie in to the grid using a pad-mounted 4-way switch (by (Electrical Provider)). One of the switches represents the utility loop in, a second switch represents the utility feed to the MOB, a third switch represents the generator tie-in to the utility loop, and the final switch represents the utility loop out. Two new 2000 kW generators will be purchased and located in the CEP (additional description to be provided in sections below). These generators will serve as the legally required essential system power source as well as the prime source in the Load Control Rate mode for both the hospital and CEP. These generators will be tied into the (Electrical Provider) utility grid (via feeders originating in the hospital's essential system paralleling gear) by way of two 3000 kVa, 480Y/277:25kV, pad-mounted, oil-filled transformers (by (Electrical Provider)). The generator outputs will tie in to the grid using a pad-mounted 5-way switch (by (Electrical Provider)). One of the switches represents the utility loop in, two switches represent the utility feeds to the CEP, and two switches represent the generator tie-ins to the utility loop.

Fire Pump Utility Service

Extend utility power from the secondary terminals of one of the 3000 kVA transformers (25kV:480Y/277V) serving the Central Energy Plant. Fire pump service feeder is to be ahead of any main breakers located in switchgear. Extend power from the transformer to the normal input terminals of the fire pump automatic transfer switch.

All protective devices are to be sized and set such that locked rotor current at the fire pump motor will not trip any protective device.

Normal Power Distribution

CEP

Extend two (2) 4000A feeders from the secondaries of two (2) pad-mounted utility transformers (anticipated 3000 kVa units by SVEC in a utility yard adjacent to CEP) to service entrance ANSI class switchgear located in the CEP. Switchgear is "main-tie-main" configuration with PLC-controlled automatic throw-over. Switchgear to utilize draw-out power circuit breakers for distribution. Assume an interrupting rating of 85K AIC.

Switchgear will feed four (4) 800-ton chillers, two (2) from each side, an 800A distribution panelboard, and a 600A motor control center. The distribution panelboard and motor control center will feed mechanical loads, the normal side of the CEP automatic transfer switches, and a house lighting panel. All electrical service equipment will be designed for future expansion capability.

Refer to the attached E3.1 for additional description/depiction of the CEP normal power distribution.

Hospital

Extend two (2) 5000A feeders from the secondaries of two (2) pad-mounted utility transformers (anticipated 4000 kVa units by SVEC in a utility yard adjacent to CEP) to service entrance ANSI class switchgear located in the CEP. Switchgear is "main-tie-main" configuration with PLC-controlled automatic throw-over. Switchgear to utilize draw-out power circuit breakers for distribution. Assume an interrupting rating of 85K AIC.

Switchgear will provide power to two distribution switchboards and one distribution panelboard, each equipped with electronic trip, molded case circuit breakers. The two distribution switchboards (2000A each) will supply power to the lower level through 2nd floor and the 3rd floor though 5th floor (as well as future 6th and 7th), respectively. A distribution panelboard (1200A) will serve the imaging equipment on the 1st floor. Two spare 2000A breakers will be provided for undetermined future needs.

The switchgear will also supply power to the normal power input of eight automatic transfer switches as described in the emergency power distribution section.

Refer to the attached E3.2 for additional description/depiction of the hospital normal power distribution.

Emergency Service

CEP and Hospital

Provide two (2) 2000kW, 480Y/277V, standby (1825kW prime) bi-fuel engine generators (Tier 2 emissions rating) inside the Central Energy Plant. Primary fuel to be number 2 diesel and alternate fuel to be natural gas under base bid. Refer to Division 15 portion of narrative for fuel oil storage system description.

Extend 4000A feeders from generator outputs to each side of 4000A emergency paralleling and synchronizing gear, ANSI class, in the CEP emergency distribution room. Paralleling switchgear is "main-tie-main" configuration with PLC-controlled automatic throw-over. Paralleling switchgear to utilize draw-out power circuit breakers for distribution. Assume an interrupting rating of 85K AIC. Paralleling gear to provide power to the emergency input of twelve (12) automatic transfer switches described below serving the CEP and hospital. These feeds represent the legally required essential electrical system for the facility.

In addition to the legally required loads, the generators will be tasked to achieve the Load Control Rate described above. Extend two (2) 4000A feeders from each side of the paralleling gear to two (2) utility transformers (anticipated 3000 kVa by (Electrical Provider)) in the utility yard adjacent to the CEP. These feeders will distribute stand-by generation to the (Electrical Provider) owned 25 kV primary loop to serve as a "prime source" in the Load Control scenario. PLC control will be provided to synchronize and parallel the generators with the utility and to analyze the load on the paralleling gear, adding/shedding loads as appropriate.

Refer to the attached E3.1 and E3.3 for additional description/depiction of the essential system distribution in the CEP and hospital.

Emergency Power Distribution

CEP

The essential system paralleling gear will supply power to the fire pump automatic transfer switch (260A), the life safety branch automatic transfer switch (70A), the Priority One equipment system automatic transfer switch (260A), and the equipment system transfer switch (800A).

- The 260A fire pump automatic transfer switch is an integral component of the fire pump controller assembly (provided by the fire pump vendor) and is in the CEP fire pump room.

- The 70A Life Safety Branch automatic transfer switch will supply a 100A lighting panel located in the emergency distribution switchgear room of the CEP.

- The 260A Priority One Equipment system automatic transfer switch will supply a 250A distribution panelboard located in the emergency distribution switchgear room of the CEP. The distribution panelboard is equipped with molded case circuit breakers that utilize electronic trip units.

- The 800A Equipment system automatic transfer switch will supply an 800A distribution panelboard located in the emergency distribution switchgear room of the CEP. The distribution panelboard is equipped with molded case circuit breakers that utilize electronic trip units.

Hospital

The essential system paralleling gear will supply power to the Life Safety Branch automatic transfer switch (400A), two Critical Branch transfer switches (1600A and 1200A), and the Equipment System transfer switches (2000A-Lower Floors, 1200A-Imaging, 1600A-Penthouse, 1600A-Penthouse, and 1200A-Elevators).

- The 400A Life Safety Branch automatic transfer switch will supply a 400A distribution panelboard located in an electrical room on the ground floor of the hospital. The distribution panelboard is equipped with molded case circuit breakers that utilize electronic trip units.
- The 1600A Critical Branch automatic transfer switch will supply a 1600A distribution switchboard located in an electrical room on the ground floor of the hospital. The distribution switchboard is equipped with molded case circuit breakers that utilize electronic trip units.
- The 1200A Critical Branch automatic transfer switch will supply a 1200A distribution panelboard located in an electrical room on the 3rd floor of the hospital. The distribution panelboard is equipped with molded case circuit breakers that utilize electronic trip units.
- The 2000A Equipment system automatic transfer switch (Lower Floors) will supply a 2000A distribution switchboard located in an electrical room on the ground floor of the hospital. The distribution switchboard is equipped with molded case circuit breakers that utilize electronic trip units.
- The 1200A Equipment system automatic transfer switch (Imaging) will supply a 1200A distribution panelboard located in an electrical room on the 1st floor of the hospital. The distribution panelboard is equipped with molded case circuit breakers that utilize electronic trip units.
- The 1600A Equipment system automatic transfer switch (Penthouse) will supply a 1600A distribution panelboard located in the penthouse on the 6th floor of the hospital. The distribution panelboard is equipped with molded case circuit breakers that utilize electronic trip units.
- The 1600A Equipment system automatic transfer switch (Penthouse) will supply a 1600A distribution panelboard located in the penthouse on the 6th floor of the hospital. The distribution panelboard is equipped with molded case circuit breakers that utilize electronic trip units.
- The 1200A Equipment system automatic transfer switch (Elevators) will supply a 1200A distribution panelboard located in the penthouse on the 6th floor of the hospital. The distribution panelboard is equipped with molded case circuit breakers that utilize electronic trip units.

Electrical Rooms

CEP

- One normal distribution switchgear room containing two double-ended main switchgear assemblies, distribution panelboards, and branch circuit panelboards.

- One emergency distribution switchgear room containing emergency paralleling gear, eleven automatic transfer switches, distribution panelboards, and branch circuit panelboards.

Hospital

- Lower Level: Three rooms containing distribution switchboards, distribution panelboards, and branch circuit panelboards. One closet containing branch circuit panelboards.

- 1st Floor: Five rooms containing distribution and branch circuit panelboards. One closet containing branch circuit panelboards

- 2nd Floor: Five rooms containing distribution and branch circuit panelboards. Four closets containing branch circuit panelboards.

- 3rd Floor: Two rooms containing distribution and branch circuit panelboards. Six closets containing branch circuit panelboards.

- 4th Floor: One room containing distribution and branch circuit panelboards. Eight closets containing branch circuit panelboards.

- 5th Floor: One room containing distribution and branch circuit panelboards. Six closets containing branch circuit panelboards.

Refer to the attached MEPT1.G-1.7 and E2.1-2.4 for electrical room locations and layouts.

Lighting

Interior Lighting

Interior building lighting will consist generally of 2x4 recessed fluorescent fixtures and compact fluorescent down lights.

In clinical spaces, back-of-house areas, and non-public corridors, fixtures will typically be 2 or 3 lamp 2x4 recessed fluorescent fixtures with prismatic acrylic lenses. In physician and business offices, fixtures will typically be 2 or 3 lamp 2x4 recessed fluorescent fixtures with 18 cell parabolic lenses. Dual level switching will be provided for 3 lamp fixtures. Operating rooms and cardiac cath labs will be provided with 6 lamp recessed fixtures with asymmetric lenses and full output Bodine emergency ballasts. Corridor lighting will generally be at 12'-0" on center. Patient rooms will be provided with a tri-mode exam light, equal to Alkco, recessed in the ceiling above the bed and dimmable compact fluorescent down lights around the perimeter of the room. Imaging equipment control rooms and physician reading rooms will be provided with dimmable compact fluorescent down lights.

Public space lighting will be as directed by the architect. In general, waiting rooms and public corridors will be provided with 2x2 recessed indirect fluorescent fixtures and decorative ADA compliant wall sconces. In general, spacing in waiting areas will be 8'-0" x 8'-0" and in corridors will be 12'-0" on center. Public space lighting will be controlled through the facility management system by way of "smart" circuit breakers. Typical color temperature for fluorescent lighting will be 4100K.

All accent, sign, display, and exterior lighting will be as directed by the architect.

All normally unoccupied areas (storage, toilets, meds, clean/soiled utility, etc.) will be provided with occupancy sensors in addition to local wall switches.

Day-lighting controls will be used where applicable in areas with a large amount of glass to minimize energy consumption during daylight hours.

Site Lighting

The site lighting is designed with cutoff style fixtures with lighting levels for site areas, landscape, and building façade lighting at or below ASHRAE Standard 90.1-2004 requirements. The fixture types and placement are designated for minimal spillover to occur at the site boundary.

Other Equipment

Electric Motors

All electric motors involved in mechanical processes (condensers, fans, pumps, compressors, etc.) meet or exceed the requirements of the Energy Policy Act of 1992 as outlined in Table 10.8, ASHRAE Standard 90.1-2004.